SIXTH EDITION

THE MATHEMATICS OF

DRUGS AND SOLUTIONS

WITH CLINICAL APPLICATIONS

Lloyd I. Richardson, Jr.
Distinguished Teaching Professor of
Education and Mathematics
University of Missouri – St. Louis

Judith K. Richardson
Associate Professor of Nursing
St. Louis Community College at
Florissant Valley

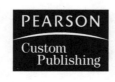

PEARSON

Custom
Publishing

unknown / 6-18 / unknown / 20.00

Ⓟ

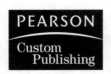

PEARSON CUSTOM PUBLISHING
75 Arlington Street, Suite 300, Boston, MA 02116
A Pearson Education Company

133651

PREFACE

It has been almost thirty years since the first publication of this text. During each revision since 1976, we have attempted to incorporate the many suggestions and constructive feedback offered by students and instructors who have used this text. This edition is no exception.

There are two important additions to this revision and each is the result of suggestions from consumers. The inclusion of learning objectives prior to each unit of study should allow students to focus on critical concepts that are presented in the chapter. Second, a chapter has been added that addresses the special needs of the geriatric client and exercises with medications such as antihypertensives that are more common with the geriatric client than with the general population.

The text continues to be a concise presentation of the mathematics associated with medications and organized in a problem-solving format. One major focus is to emphasize the development of a math strategy to be used to solve all problems presented in the text. The learner is guided through the step-by-step process of identifying and solving a problem. The guided examples develop the learner's critical thinking and problem-solving skills by providing maximal guidance in the first example, less guidance in the next example, and selectively removing guidance until the learner can reason through the problem without any prompting. For this reason it is essential that the learner work through the guided example step-by-step and check the correctness of each step before continuing in the text. Answers to the guided examples have been placed at the end of each chapter to facilitate checking examples.

Space has been provided in the text for students to work the exercises and guided examples. This will facilitate later review and the text will serve as a resource to the learner.

We would like to acknowledge the following people for their assistance with this book.

David A. Palkovich, MA
Professor of Mathematics
Oklahoma City Community College
Oklahoma City, Oklahoma
Math content reviewer

Eng Teng Yap
Research Associate
University of Missouri-St. Louis
Computer Programmer

Sister Theresa Monaghan, RN, BSN, MA
Department of Nursing
Gwynedd Mercy College
Gwynedd Valley, Pennsylvania
Drugs & Solutions Practice Disk reviewer

Michael J. Reddy
Freelance Artist
Cartoons

TO THE STUDENT

This text begins with a review of basic math concepts. The review was written primarily for the student who has been out of school for a number of years and usually has some math anxiety and may be apprehensive about succeeding in a nursing major. It is written in a non-threatening style and provides immediate and positive feedback to reinforce the learner at each step. The review is not intended for all learners, and those with basic mathematics skills should omit this unit and begin with chapters that apply these math skills directly to medication calculations.

All sections provide numerous practice sets, and the inclusion of learning objectives at the beginning of each chapter should focus attention on major concepts. The special needs of geriatric clients are addressed in Chapter 8. The text is designed to provide guided examples that begin with maximum guidance in the first example, less guidance in the next example, and removes guidance until the learner call reason through the problem without prompting. Space is provided so all work can be done in the text and it will later serve as a resource when reviewing.

CONTENTS

THE MATHEMATICS OF

DRUGS AND SOLUTIONS

WITH CLINICAL APPLICATIONS

Unit 1 consists of Chapter 1, Mathematics Review, and Chapter 2, Systems of Measure. The intent in this unit is to provide maximal practice with the mathematical operations and measurement systems without focusing on their applications to nursing. The targeted applications to nursing are established in the next unit.

Manipulation of the mathematical operations and measurement systems are introduced, refined, and practiced. The intent in Unit 1 is to develop proficiency in utilizing the mathematical operations and understanding the measurement systems together with changing measurement values from one system to another.

1 MATHEMATICS REVIEW

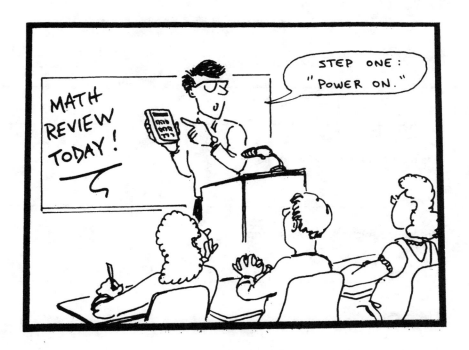

CHAPTER OBJECTIVES

- Utilize pretest to assess level of mathematics competencies
- Identify the two numeration systems
- Understand the basic operations of fractions, decimals, and percentages
- Solve problems using ratio and proportion

INTRODUCTION

This chapter reviews the basic mathematics concepts the nurse needs to compute dosages. Each concept is later utilized as an integral part of a computation involved in the daily routine of the practicing nurse.

A pretest is provided so that you can assess your need for a review of basic mathematics. Students scoring 85% or higher on the pretest are advised to begin with Chapter 2.

This chapter assumes very little prior knowledge and offers maximal guidance in the instruction. The purpose is to establish reasoning patterns and procedures for students who have difficulty with mathematical processes. Numerous exercises are provided on each topic.

When you have finished this chapter, take the posttest to see how much progress you have made. Answers to the pretest, posttest, and exercises are given at the back of this book.

Pretest

Express the following Hindu-Arabic numerals as Roman numerals:

1. 17 = _____   **2.** 342 = _____

3. 3 = _____   **4.** 25 = _____

Express the following Roman numerals as Hindu-Arabic numerals:

5. XVI = _____   **6.** CCLVII = _____

7. ix = _____   **8.** viii = _____

9. In the fraction $\frac{17}{32}$, the numerator is _____

Are the fractions equal (yes or no)?

10. $\frac{3}{8}, \frac{9}{24}$ _____   **11.** $\frac{5}{9}, \frac{18}{36}$ _____

Reduce the fractions to lowest terms:

12. $\frac{9}{48}$ = _____   **13.** $\frac{25}{75}$ = _____

14. $\frac{21}{28}$ = _____   **15.** $\frac{11}{56}$ = _____

Change the mixed numbers to fractions:

16. $4\frac{2}{3}$ _____   **17.** $2\frac{1}{8}$ _____

18. $13\frac{3}{10}$ _____

Perform the indicated operation, expressing the answer in the simplest forms:

19. $\frac{3}{8} \times \frac{4}{5}$ = _____   **20.** $\frac{5}{6} \times \frac{11}{13}$ = _____

21. $3\frac{1}{3} \times \frac{2}{5}$ = _____   **22.** $\frac{3}{8} \div \frac{4}{5}$ = _____

23. 16 ÷ 3   = _____   **24.** $\dfrac{\frac{1}{7}}{\frac{3}{8}}$ = _____

25. $5\,\overline{\smash{)}3}$ = _____   **26.** 2.137 + 1.91 = _____

27. $5.54 - 1.02$ = _____   **28.** 6.35×1.118 = _____

29. 0.074×1.385 = _____   **30.** $8.165 \div 0.15$ = _____

31. $0.013 \div 0.4$ = _____

Change the percents to decimals:

32. 5% = _____   **33.** 0.6% = _____

34. 89% = _____

Change the decimals to percents:

35. 0.46 = _____   **36.** 0.03 = _____

37. 0.175 = _____

Solve for the value of x:

38. $\frac{7}{8} = \frac{x}{12}$ _____   **39.** $\frac{x}{10} = \frac{3}{5}$ _____

40. $\frac{x}{7} = \frac{3}{11}$ _____

NUMBER SYSTEMS

The modern nurse is faced with two numeration systems and must know how to use them both. The two systems are the *Hindu-Arabic* system and the *Roman* system.

The Hindu-Arabic System

The Hindu-Arabic system consists of the symbols (often called digits)

$$0 \quad 1 \quad 2 \quad 3 \quad 4 \quad 5 \quad 6 \quad 7 \quad 8 \quad 9$$

This system is the one with which we are most familiar. In this system, a number is depicted by arranging the digits in a prescribed manner. In the arrangement of the digits, the relative place the digit occupies provides a key to its value. Thus the Hindu-Arabic system is a *place-value* system.

EXAMPLE 1.1

342 means 3 hundreds, 4 tens, and 2 units. That is, $342 = 3(100) + 4(10) + 2$, so that the position the symbol occupies in writing the number provides a key to the value of the number. Consider the number 423. 423 means 4 hundreds, 2 tens, 3 units; that is, $432 = 4(100) + 2(10) + 3$.

Although the same symbols (2, 3, and 4) are used in expressing the numbers 342 and 432, the arrangement of the symbols provides the key to the value of the number. This system should be recognized as the standard system that has been used for years. Let us now look at the Roman system.

The Roman System

The Roman system uses the symbols

$$I \quad V \quad X \quad L \quad C \quad D \quad M$$

Each symbol represents a number:

I = 1	L = 50	M = 1000
V = 5	C = 100	
X = 10	D = 500	

Certain principles are observed in the Roman system to lessen the necessity to repeat symbols so often in writing a number. The symbols V, L, and D are not repeated because there are symbols for 10, 100, and 1000. However, symbols are grouped together to form numbers. To express symbols in the Roman system, certain rules must be followed.

RULE 1: Symbols may be repeated to form a number, but a symbol may never be repeated more than 3 times in succession.

EXAMPLE 1.2

Correct: III is three.
           XXX is thirty.
           XX is twenty.
           CCC is three hundred.
           II is two.

Incorrect: VVV is not used for 15. Since we have a symbol for ten (X), the number 15 will be written   XV

                $\nearrow$ $\nwarrow$
             10   5

DDD is not used for 1500. Since we have a symbol for 1000 (M), the number 1500 should be written   MD

             $\nearrow$ $\nwarrow$
          1000   500

RULE 2: When a symbol is followed by a symbol (or symbols) representing a lesser value, the values are added to obtain the value the symbols represent.

To evaluate the value of VII, reason as follows:

VII   The symbols II are of lesser value than the symbol V; thus VII represents 5 plus 2 equals 7. We added the values 5 and 2 because the symbols satisfy Rule 2. *Read the rule again.*

EXAMPLE 1.3*

   XV represents 10 plus 5 equals 15.
   XVI represents 10 plus 5 plus 1 equals 16.
   CV represents 100 plus 5 equals 105.
   CXXI represents 100 plus 20 plus 1 equals 121.

Complete the following:

   VIII represents _____ plus _____ equals _____ .
   XII represents _____ plus _____ equals _____ .
   XXV represents _____ .
   XXXVII represents _____ plus _____ plus _____ equals _____ .

---

*Answers to examples appear on pages 43-44.

RULE 3: When a symbol of lesser value precedes a symbol of greater value, the smaller value must be subtracted from the larger to obtain the value the symbols represent.

EXAMPLE 1.4

IV   A symbol of lesser value precedes a symbol of greater value; thus IV represents a 5 minus 1, or 4; (5 − 1 = 4).
XL represents 50 − 10 = 40.
CM represents 1000 − 100 = 900.

Complete the following:

CD represents _____ minus _____ equals _____ .
IX represents _____ − _____ = _____ .
XC represents _____ .
IV represents _____ .

RULE 4: When a symbol represents a lesser value than the value of either of the symbols it appears between, the subtraction rule (Rule 3) takes precedence. The value resulting from the subtraction is added to the value of the first symbol.

EXAMPLE 1.5

XIV The symbol of lesser value, I, appears between symbols representing greater values, X and V. Thus, by Rule 4, 1 is subtracted from 5 and then the result is added to 10.

XIV represents 10 plus (5 − 1) = 14.
XIX represents 10 plus (10 − 1) = 19.
XXIV represents 20 plus (5 − 1) = 24.
CXLVI represents 100 plus 40 plus 6 = 146.
100 + (50 − 10) + (5 + 1) = 100 + 40 + 6 = 146.

In the hospital you will encounter Roman numerals when prescriptions or dosages are written in the apothecaries' system of measures. (This system will be discussed in detail in Chapter 2.) Here we need only note that when Roman numerals are used for prescriptions or dosages, the symbols are written as lowercase letters. The usual symbols are

Roman numerals	Hindu-Arabic equivalent
i	1
v	5
x	10
l	50
c	100

The use of both capital and lowercase letters to represent Roman numerals necessitates two parts to the following exercise set. The mathematics section focuses on the Roman system, where capital letters are used; the drug section focuses on the lowercase letters.

Exercise 1

Express the following Roman numerals as Hindu-Arabic numerals:

1. III   = _____

2. XII   = _____

3. XXV = _____

4. XIX   = _____

  5. XL = _____   6. LVII = _____

  7. XX = _____   8. XLVII = _____

  9. XXIX = _____   10. CC   = _____

Express the following Hindu-Arabic numerals as Roman numerals:

11. 5   = _____   12. 10 = _____

13. 15 = _____   14. 47 = _____

15. 7   = _____   16. 28 = _____

17. 39 = _____   18. 54 = _____

19. 176 = _____   20. 721 = _____

For additional practice, fill in the blanks with the correct Hindu-Arabic or Roman numerals as required:

21. VI   = _____   22. XXV   = _____

23. XXVIII = _____   24. XXXIV = _____

25. LXXIX = _____   26. IV   = _____

27. XC   = _____   28. XCV   = _____

29. XI   = _____   30. II   = _____

31. 64   = _____   32. 85   = _____

33. 19   = _____   34. 23   = _____

35. 11   = _____   36. 93   = _____

37. 41   = _____   38. 78   = _____

39. 55   = _____   40. 119   = _____

Fill in the blanks with the correct Hindu-Arabic numerals:

41. i   = _____   42. iii = _____

43. ix   = _____   44. v   = _____

45. xiii = _____   46. vii = _____

47. iv   = _____   48. viii = _____

49. xi   = _____   50. xix = _____

FRACTIONS

Fractions are important in the computation of drug dosages. Familiarity with multiplication and division of fractions will allow the nurse to concentrate on the proper procedure of drug administration instead of spending unnecessary time puzzling over the arithmetic. Only computations that are actually used in calculating dosages will be reviewed.

The word fraction is derived from the Latin word *fractus,* meaning broken. Fractions were first thought of as broken numbers. Indeed, a fraction is a number that represents part of a whole unit. A fraction consists of two parts, the numerator and the denominator:

$$\frac{a}{b} \qquad \begin{array}{l} a \text{ is the numerator} \\ b \text{ is the denominator} \end{array}$$

The denominator tells the number of equal parts into which the whole is separated. The numerator tells how many of the equal parts are being considered:

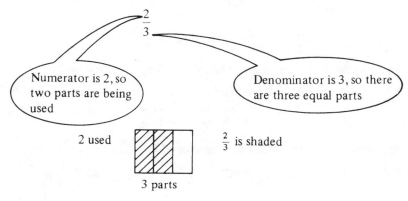

The fraction is two thirds. Two parts are being considered from the whole that is divided into three parts.

EXAMPLE 1.6

$\dfrac{3}{8}$ The numerator of the fraction is 3.
The denominator of the fraction is 8.

$\dfrac{5}{7}$ The numerator of the fraction is _____ .
The denominator of the fraction is _____ .

$\dfrac{4}{5}$ Numerator is _____ ; denominator is _____ .

How can you determine when two fractions are equal? For instance, fractions $\frac{1}{2}$ and $\frac{2}{4}$ are equal fractions since each fraction represents half (see Figure 1-1).

Figure 1-1

From Figure 1-1 it is obvious that $\frac{1}{2}$ and $\frac{2}{4}$ have the same amount of shaded area. This means that they represent the same part of the unit but have different names. Just as $1 + 4$, $3 + 2$, $4 + 1$, and $0 + 5$ all name the number 5, the fractions $\frac{1}{2}$ and $\frac{2}{4}$ are names for the same number. Therefore they are called equal.

Since the fractions $\frac{1}{2}$ and $\frac{2}{4}$ are equal, let us inspect them to see what characteristics will show the equality without having to rely on a drawing. Notice that if the numerator of the fraction $\frac{1}{2}$ is multiplied by 2, we get the numerator of the fraction $\frac{2}{4}$:

$$\frac{1 \times \boxed{2} \rightarrow \boxed{2}}{2 \qquad\qquad 4}$$

Now multiply the denominator of the fraction $\frac{1}{2}$ by the same number, 2:

$$\frac{1}{2 \times \boxed{2} \rightarrow \frac{2}{4}}$$

We get 4, the value of the denominator of the fraction $\frac{2}{4}$, that is,

$$\frac{1 \times 2}{2 \times 2} = \frac{2}{4}$$

Multiplying both the numerator and denominator of the fraction $\frac{1}{2}$ by the same number, 2, yields an equal fraction, $\frac{2}{4}$.

> **RULE:** If both the numerator and denominator of a fraction are multiplied by the same number, the resulting fraction is equal to the original fraction.

> **ALTERNATIVE:** Two fractions are equal if one fraction can be obtained from the other by multiplying both the numerator and denominator of the first fraction by the same number.

For example, are the fractions $\frac{2}{3}$ and $\frac{4}{6}$ equal?

Begin by asking yourself, "What must the numerator of the fraction $\frac{2}{3}$ be multiplied by in order to obtain the numerator of the fraction $\frac{4}{6}$?"

$$\frac{2}{3} \times \boxed{} \longrightarrow \frac{4}{6}$$

The answer is obviously 2 since 2 times 2 is 4:

$$\frac{2}{3} \times \frac{2}{2} = \frac{4}{6}$$

Check the value you just obtained, 2, to see if multiplying the denominator of the fraction $\frac{2}{3}$ by 2 will yield the denominator of the fraction $\frac{4}{6}$.

Certainly it does since 3 times 2 equals 6. The two fractions $\frac{2}{3}$ and $\frac{4}{6}$ are equal because multiplying both numerator and denominator of the fraction $\frac{2}{3}$ by the same number, 2, yields the fraction $\frac{4}{6}$.

Are the fractions $\frac{4}{5}$ and $\frac{12}{15}$ equal? What number must the numerator of the fraction $\frac{4}{5}$ be multiplied by to get the numerator of the fraction $\frac{12}{15}$?

$$\frac{4}{5} \times \boxed{?} \rightarrow \frac{12}{15}$$

The 4 must be multiplied by 3 to get 12. Now check to see if 3 times the denominator of $\frac{4}{5}$ is the same as the denominator of $\frac{12}{15}$.

Yes, 5 times 3 is 15.
Are the fractions $\frac{7}{11}$ and $\frac{21}{33}$ equal?

$$\frac{4 \times 3}{5 \times \boxed{3}} = \frac{12}{15}$$

$$\frac{7}{11} \times \overset{3}{?} \rightarrow \frac{21}{33}$$

$$\frac{7}{11} \times \overset{3}{?} \longrightarrow \frac{21}{33}$$

The numerator must be multiplied by 3.

$$\frac{7 \times 3}{11 \times \boxed{3}} = \frac{21}{33}$$

$$\boxed{11 \times 3 = ? \atop 11 \times 3 = 33}$$

Thus the two fractions are equal.
Are the fractions $\frac{3}{8}$ and $\frac{15}{32}$ equal?

$$\frac{3}{8} \times \boxed{?} \rightarrow \frac{15}{32}$$

$$\frac{3}{8} \times \boxed{5} \rightarrow \frac{15}{32}$$

$$\frac{3 \times 5}{8 \times \boxed{5}} \overset{?}{=} \frac{15}{32} \qquad \text{No! } 8 \times 5 = 40$$

So

$$\frac{3 \times 5}{8 \times 5} \text{ does not equal } \frac{15}{32}$$

and the fractions are not equal fractions.

One of the more important implications of the fact that when the numerator and denominator of a fraction are multiplied by the same number, the resultant fraction is equal to the original fraction is that we can use it to reduce fractions to lowest terms. Consider the fraction $\frac{16}{40}$, which can be expressed as

$$\frac{16}{40} = \frac{2 \times 8}{5 \times 8}$$

Draw the line all the way as a reminder that one 8 is multiplied by the numerator while the second 8 is multiplied by the denominator

or 2 times 8 divided by 5 times 8. By the reasoning used in the previous examples, the fraction $\frac{2}{5}$ is equal to the fraction $\frac{16}{40}$. In many cases it is desirable to rename fractions (such as $\frac{16}{40}$ renamed $\frac{2}{5}$) so that the computation is easier (using 2 and 5 is easier than using 16 and 40).

One procedure for reducing fractions is cancellation. To use cancellation, first find a number common to both the numerator and the denominator (in the above example 8 is common to both the numerator and the denominator). Second, cancel the member that appears in a product in both the numerator and the denominator. Third, use the remaining numerator and denominator as the renamed fraction. To work the above problem proceed as follows:

$$\frac{16}{40} = \frac{2 \times 8}{5 \times 8} = \frac{2 \times \cancel{8}}{5 \times \cancel{8}} = \frac{2}{5}$$

Cancel the value 8 because it is common to both the numerator and denominator

RULE: If both the numerator and the denominator of a fraction are multiplied by the same number, the number may be cancelled without changing the value of the fraction. (Answers should always be expressed in lowest terms, where no number is a factor of both the numerator and the denominator.)

EXAMPLE 1.7

$\frac{18}{48} = \frac{3 \times 6}{8 \times 6}$, so cancel the 6 leaving $\frac{3}{8}$

In mathematical form

$$\frac{18}{48} = \frac{3 \times \cancel{6}}{8 \times \cancel{6}} = \frac{3}{8}$$

$$\frac{40}{55} = \frac{8 \times \cancel{5}}{11 \times \cancel{5}} = \frac{8}{11}$$

Complete the following:

$$\frac{15}{50} = \frac{3 \times \boxed{}}{10 \times 5} = \frac{\boxed{}}{10}$$

$$\frac{28}{64} = \frac{7 \times \boxed{}}{\boxed{} \times \boxed{}} = \frac{7}{\boxed{}}$$

$$\frac{32}{80} = \frac{2 \times \boxed{}}{\boxed{} \times 16} = \frac{2}{\boxed{}}$$

$$\frac{54}{66} = \frac{\boxed{} \times \boxed{}}{11 \times \boxed{}} = \frac{\boxed{}}{\boxed{}}$$

$$\frac{21}{35} = \frac{3 \times \boxed{}}{\boxed{} \times 7} = \frac{3}{\boxed{}}$$

$$\frac{8}{32} = \frac{\boxed{} \times \boxed{}}{4 \times \boxed{}} = \frac{\boxed{}}{\boxed{}}$$

Exercise 2

Reduce the following fractions by using the cancellation rule given above:

1. $\frac{8}{20}$

2. $\frac{18}{32}$

3. $\frac{21}{24}$

4. $\frac{30}{35}$

5. $\frac{9}{12}$

6. $\frac{20}{30}$

7. $\frac{4}{8}$

8. $\frac{5}{25}$

9. $\frac{100}{200}$

10. $\frac{18}{72}$

Continue as above for extra practice:

11. $\frac{6}{12}$

12. $\frac{2}{10}$

13. $\frac{5}{15}$

14. $\frac{150}{200}$

15. $\frac{9}{48}$

16. $\frac{15}{48}$

17. $\frac{7}{28}$

18. $\frac{24}{30}$

19. $\frac{11}{33}$

20. $\frac{12}{32}$

Types of Fractions

Basically there are two types of fractions. Each type may occur in drug and solution problems. Each type is presented here with examples, so that you can refer back to this explanation.

1. *Common fractions* The numerator and the denominator are both whole numbers:

$$\frac{11}{16}, \frac{1}{7}, \text{ and } \frac{3}{8} \text{ are common fractions}$$

a. *Proper fractions* The numerator is smaller than the denominator:

$\frac{3}{4}$ is a proper fraction because the numerator (3) is smaller than the denominator (4)

b. *Improper fractions* The numerator is larger than the denominator:

$\frac{8}{5}$ is an improper fraction because the numerator (8) is larger than the denominator (5)

2. *Complex fractions* A fraction where the numerator or the denominator (or both) is itself a fraction:

$$\frac{\frac{3}{8}}{\frac{1}{2}} \text{ is a complex fraction}$$

$$\frac{\frac{4}{5}}{2} \text{ is a complex fraction}$$

$$\frac{3}{\frac{1}{8}} \text{ is a complex fraction}$$

Notice that the main division line (separating the numerator and denominator) is an extended line so that confusion is avoided. For example,

$$\frac{2}{\frac{3}{4}}$$

might be thought of as 2 divided by the fraction $\frac{3}{4}$. Also it could be the fraction $\frac{2}{3}$ divided by 4. Which is correct? No one knows! If the fraction is written

$$\frac{2}{\frac{3}{4}}$$

it can be said that the complex fraction is 2 divided by the fraction $\frac{3}{4}$. It is very important that the main division line be an extended line!

A *mixed number* is a whole number combined with a fraction. The number $2\frac{3}{4}$ is a mixed number and is read two and three-fourths.

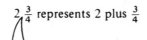

$2\frac{3}{4}$ represents 2 plus $\frac{3}{4}$

This is a case where multiplication is not implied. That is, $2\frac{3}{4}$ *does not* mean $2 \times \frac{3}{4}$; instead adjacent positioning means add (+) in this case

Since 2 is the same as $\frac{8}{4}$,

$$2 + \frac{3}{4} = \frac{8}{4} + \frac{3}{4} = \frac{11}{4}$$

so the mixed number $2\frac{3}{4}$ is the same as the fraction $\frac{11}{4}$. A simple method for converting a mixed number to a fraction form is as follows:

$$2\frac{3}{4} = \frac{2 \times 4 + 3}{4} = \frac{8 + 3}{4} = \frac{11}{4}$$

RULE: To change a mixed number to a fraction, multiply the denominator of the fraction by the whole number and add this to the numerator of the fraction. This yields the numerator of the equivalent fraction. The denominator of the equivalent fraction is the same as the denominator of the original fraction.

For the mixed number $2\frac{3}{4}$, multiply the denominator (4) by the whole number (2) and add this to the numerator of the fraction (3). This yields the numerator of the equivalent fraction (11). The denominator of the equivalent fraction is the same as the denominator of the original fraction (4). Thus

$$2\frac{3}{4} = \frac{11}{4}$$

For the mixed number $7\frac{2}{5}$,

$$7\frac{2}{5} = \frac{7 \times 5 + 2}{5} = \frac{35 + 2}{5} = \frac{37}{5}$$

The mixed number $7\frac{2}{5}$ is converted to fraction form by multiplying 7 by 5 and adding 2 to get the numerator; 7 times 5 is 35; adding 2 gives 37. The denominator of the fraction remains 5.

EXAMPLE 1.8

Complete the following:

$$5\frac{3}{8} = \frac{\boxed{} \times 8 + \boxed{}}{\boxed{}} = \frac{}{} = \frac{}{}$$

$$3\frac{5}{11} = \frac{\boxed{} \times \boxed{} + \boxed{}}{11} = \frac{}{11} = \frac{}{11}$$

$$2\frac{7}{9} = \frac{\boxed{} \times \boxed{} + \boxed{}}{\boxed{}} = \frac{}{}$$

Exercise 3

Convert the following mixed numbers to improper fractions:

1. $2\frac{3}{4}$

2. $1\frac{1}{2}$

3. $4\frac{1}{8}$

4. $1\frac{3}{10}$

5. $3\frac{5}{8}$

6. $12\frac{3}{5}$

7. $1\frac{8}{10}$

8. $6\frac{1}{3}$

9. $5\frac{2}{5}$

10. $100\frac{5}{7}$

Adding and Subtracting Fractions

This section provides rules for adding and subtracting fractions so that systematic computation can be accomplished without guesswork.

Consider adding $\frac{2}{5}$ and $\frac{1}{5}$.

$$\frac{2}{5} + \frac{1}{5} = ?$$

The fraction $\frac{2}{5}$ means 2 parts of a unit that has been divided into 5 equal parts. Thus $\frac{2}{5}$ is

and $\frac{1}{5}$ is

Joining the shaded areas together yields

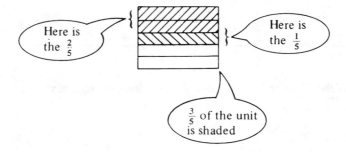

$\frac{3}{5}$, that is, 3 parts used in a total of 5. Thus

$$\frac{2}{5} + \frac{1}{5} = \frac{3}{5}$$

When the denominators are the same (in this case, both fractions have a denominator of 5), the sum is obtained by adding the numerators and placing the sum over the denominator:

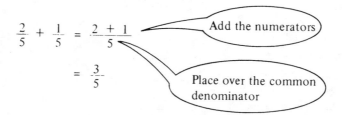

The fractions to be added may not always have like denominators. Consider

$$\frac{1}{2} + \frac{1}{3} = ?$$

Recall from a previous section that

$$\frac{1}{2} = \frac{3}{6} \text{ also } \frac{1}{3} = \frac{2}{6}$$

so

$$\frac{1}{2} + \frac{1}{3} = \frac{3}{6} + \frac{2}{6} = \frac{3 + 2}{6} = \frac{5}{6}$$

Replacing $\frac{1}{2}$ by equivalent $\frac{3}{6}$

Replacing $\frac{1}{3}$ by equivalent $\frac{2}{6}$

The sum becomes $\frac{5}{6}$.

In this case the number 6 is the common denominator. A *common denominator* is a number that each of the denominators will divide. For the problem

$$\frac{1}{4} + \frac{2}{3} = ?$$

the denominators are 4 and 3. The least number they will both divide is 12. Thus

$$\frac{1}{4} + \frac{2}{3} =$$

$$\frac{3}{12} + \frac{8}{12} = \frac{3 + 8}{12} = \frac{11}{12}$$

Convert each fraction to an equivalent fraction with a denominator of 12

RULE: To add fractions

1. Find a common denominator.
2. Convert each fraction to an equivalent fraction with the common denominator.
3. Add the numerators and place them over the common denominator.

EXAMPLE 1.9

$$\frac{2}{5} + \frac{1}{6} = ?$$

1. The common denominator is _____ .

2. Equivalent fraction for $\frac{2}{5}$ = _____ .

3. Equivalent fraction for $\frac{1}{6}$ = _____ .

4. Find the sum.

Subtracting fractions involves the same reasoning except that the numerators are subtracted rather than added. In the problem

$$\frac{2}{3} - \frac{1}{4} = ?$$

the least common denominator is 12.

$$\frac{2}{3} - \frac{1}{4} \text{ becomes } \frac{8}{12} - \frac{3}{12}$$

which equals

$$\frac{8 - 3}{12} = \frac{5}{12}$$

Once the fractions involving the common denominator are obtained, the numerators are subtracted. The denominator of the resulting fraction is the common denominator.

RULE: To subtract fractions:

1. Find a common denominator.
2. Convert each fraction to an equivalent fraction with the common denominator.
3. Subtract the numerator of the equivalent fractions and place the difference over the common denominator.

Exercise 4

Use the rules to solve the following:

1. $\frac{3}{7} + \frac{2}{7} =$

2. $\frac{5}{8} - \frac{3}{8} =$

3. $\frac{1}{8} + \frac{1}{2} =$

4. $\frac{4}{9} - \frac{1}{3} =$

5. $\frac{4}{5} + \frac{1}{3} =$ **6.** $\frac{7}{11} - \frac{1}{2} =$

7. $\frac{3}{8} + \frac{5}{6} =$ **8.** $\frac{8}{9} - \frac{5}{12} =$

9. $1\frac{2}{5} + 3\frac{1}{4} =$ **10.** $2\frac{1}{6} - 1\frac{1}{2} =$

Multiplication of Fractions

RULE: When multiplying two fractions, the result is obtained by multiplying the numerators and dividing by the product of the denominators; i.e., numerator times numerator and denominator times denominator.

EXAMPLE 1.10

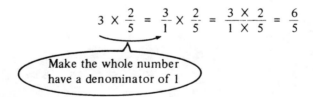

$$\frac{3}{4} \times \frac{5}{7} = \frac{3 \times 5}{4 \times 7} = \frac{15}{28}$$

$$\frac{2}{9} \times \frac{4}{5} = \frac{2 \times 4}{9 \times 5} = \frac{8}{45}$$

$$\frac{1}{64} \times \frac{3}{4} = \frac{1 \times 3}{64 \times 4} = \frac{3}{256}$$

A whole number such as 3 may be written as the fraction $\frac{3}{1}$, so that when multiplying a whole number by a fraction, say 3 by $\frac{2}{5}$,

$$3 \times \frac{2}{5} = \frac{3}{1} \times \frac{2}{5} = \frac{3 \times 2}{1 \times 5} = \frac{6}{5}$$

Make the whole number have a denominator of 1

the whole number 3 is replaced by the fraction $\frac{3}{1}$ and the rule for multiplying fractions can be applied. Alternatively, you can remember that when multiplying a whole number by a fraction, the whole number is multiplied by the numerator of the fraction

$$6 \times \frac{5}{7} = \frac{6 \times 5}{7} = \frac{30}{7}$$

or

$$6 \times \frac{5}{7} = \frac{6}{1} \times \frac{5}{7} = \frac{6 \times 5}{1 \times 7} = \frac{30}{7}$$

Notice the answers are identical

A mixed number should be written as a fraction before multiplying

$$2\frac{1}{4} \times \frac{3}{7} = \frac{9}{4} \times \frac{3}{7} = \frac{27}{28}$$

Exercise 5

Multiply the following fractions and reduce to lowest terms:

1. $\frac{2}{3} \times \frac{5}{7}$ 2. $\frac{3}{4} \times \frac{1}{2}$

3. $\frac{5}{6} \times \frac{3}{8}$ 4. $\frac{7}{9} \times \frac{2}{3}$

5. $\frac{1}{8} \times \frac{4}{5}$ 6. $\frac{3}{2} \times \frac{4}{5}$

7. $3 \times \frac{1}{8}$ 8. $4 \times \frac{4}{5}$

9. $2\frac{1}{2} \times \frac{3}{8}$ 10. $3\frac{1}{5} \times \frac{5}{8}$

Continue as above for extra practice:

11. $\frac{8}{9} \times \frac{5}{6}$ 12. $1\frac{1}{25} \times \frac{4}{10}$

13. $\frac{3}{7} \times \frac{21}{22}$ 14. $2\frac{3}{10} \times 1\frac{1}{5}$

15. $\frac{22}{36} \times \frac{6}{11}$ 16. $9 \times \frac{2}{3}$

17. $7 \times 7\frac{1}{2}$ 18. $18 \times \frac{1}{6}$

19. $4\frac{1}{5} \times \frac{1}{5}$ 20. $3\frac{1}{13} \times \frac{17}{20}$

Division of Fractions

The rule for division of fractions depends on understanding how to multiply fractions.

Look for a moment at the mathematical meaning of the word *invert*. The word *invert* means to interchange the numerator and denominator of the given fraction. If the fraction $\frac{3}{8}$ is inverted, the result is the fraction $\frac{8}{3}$. Inverting $\frac{4}{5}$ makes it $\frac{5}{4}$.

RULE: When dividing two fractions, the result is obtained by inverting the fraction in the denominator, then multiplying the numerator fraction by the inverted denominator fraction.

EXAMPLE 1.11

Divide the following fractions:

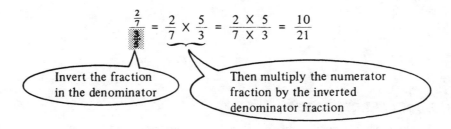

$$\frac{\frac{2}{7}}{\frac{3}{5}} = \frac{2}{7} \times \frac{5}{3} = \frac{2 \times 5}{7 \times 3} = \frac{10}{21}$$

Invert the fraction in the denominator

Then multiply the numerator fraction by the inverted denominator fraction

$$\frac{\frac{2}{3}}{\frac{5}{7}} = \frac{2}{3} \times \frac{7}{5} = \frac{2 \times 7}{3 \times 5} = \frac{14}{15}$$

$$\frac{5}{\frac{3}{8}} = 5 \times \frac{8}{3} = \frac{5 \times 8}{3} = \frac{40}{3}$$

$$\frac{\frac{2}{9}}{11} = \frac{\frac{2}{9}}{\frac{11}{1}} = \frac{2}{9} \times \frac{1}{11} = \frac{2 \times 1}{9 \times 11} = \frac{2}{99}$$

Exercise 6

Reduce answers to the simplest form:

1. $\frac{3}{4} \div \frac{2}{3}$

2. $\frac{5}{8} \div \frac{10}{16}$

3. $\frac{4}{7} \div \frac{8}{9}$

4. $3 \div \frac{1}{2}$

Continue as above for extra practice:

5. $\frac{9}{16} \div 3$

6. $\frac{7}{16} \div \frac{7}{8}$

7. $\frac{1}{75} \div \frac{6}{25}$

8. $\frac{1}{12} \div \frac{3}{24}$

9. $\frac{1}{4} \div \frac{7}{20}$

10. $2\frac{3}{4} \div 6\frac{1}{2}$

11. $230 \div 4\frac{1}{2}$

12. $\frac{1}{50} \div \frac{1}{10}$

13. $\frac{2}{9} \div \frac{3}{12}$

14. $\frac{7}{3} \div \frac{2}{21}$

15. $2\frac{1}{2} \div 5$

16. $\frac{1}{100} \div 8$

17. $\frac{1}{64} \div \frac{1}{8}$

18. $\frac{1}{8} \div \frac{1}{64}$

19. $1\frac{1}{3} \div \frac{1}{10}$

20. $\frac{11}{69} \div \frac{22}{36}$

DECIMALS AND PERCENTAGES

Working with decimal numbers often seems mysterious and without rules of order. Actually decimal numbers obey strict rules and are useful because they allow a compact notation for numbers.

A decimal number consists of a decimal point and numbers to both the left and right of the decimal point. Just as whole numbers have positions such as units, tens, hundreds, etc., decimal numbers expand this idea and name points to the right of the decimal point.

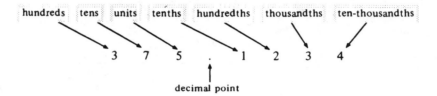

Let us investigate positions to the right of the decimal point and identify what each position means. Consider 5.1, which is read as five and one-tenth. This means $5 + \frac{1}{10}$ or, as we discussed previously, $5\frac{1}{10}$. Extending work with decimals, 5.12, which is read as five and twelve-hundredths, means

$$5 + \frac{1}{10} + \frac{2}{100} \text{ or } 5 + \frac{12}{100}$$

What decimal number would represent the number

$$7 + \frac{9}{10} + \frac{6}{100} + \frac{3}{1000}$$

The number would be 7.963 since there are 9 tenths, 6 hundredths, and 3 thousandths.

Read the number 4.35 as four and thirty-five hundredths. To read a decimal number, look at the last number to the right of the decimal point. Here the digit 5 is in the hundredths column, so the number to the right of the decimal is read as one number (thirty-five) followed by the appropriate classification (hundredths).

Earlier it was stated that 4.35 represents

$$4 + \frac{3}{10} + \frac{5}{100}$$

and now we are implying that 4.35 is

$$4 + \frac{35}{100}$$

Are these the same? Consider $4 + \frac{3}{10} + \frac{5}{100}$

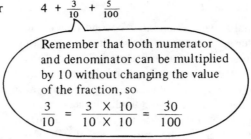

Remember that both numerator and denominator can be multiplied by 10 without changing the value of the fraction, so

$$\frac{3}{10} = \frac{3 \times 10}{10 \times 10} = \frac{30}{100}$$

and replace $\frac{3}{10}$ by $\frac{30}{100}$, obtaining

$$4 + \frac{30}{100} + \frac{5}{100} \text{ and this is } 4 + \frac{35}{100}$$

Yes, the representations are equal.

Whole numbers are actually decimal numbers. A number like 11 is a decimal number, but because there is no decimal portion to the number, it is understood that the decimal falls to the right of the units digit. Thus

$$11 = 11. \text{ and } 7410 = 7410.$$

Notice that 11 may be written as 11.000 and have exactly the same value. As many zeros as one wishes or needs may be added to the right of the decimal without altering the value of the number. Thus

$$254 = 254. = 254.00 = 254.00000$$

A fraction can be changed to a decimal number by dividing the numerator of the fraction by the denominator of the fraction; that is, $\frac{1}{2}$ can be represented as 0.5 since

$$\frac{1}{2} \text{ is } \quad 2\overline{\smash{)}1.0} \quad \begin{array}{l} \text{Numerator (1.0)} \\ \text{divided by the} \\ \text{denominator (2)} \end{array}$$

$$\begin{array}{r} 0.5 \\ \underline{1\ 0} \\ 0 \end{array}$$

Notice that the 1 in the numerator was replaced by 1.0 and the decimal point in the answer is placed directly above the decimal point in the dividend (the number to be divided).

To convert $\frac{15}{32}$ to a fraction, divide 15 by 32. Remember the decimal point is just to the right of the 5 in 15 since the decimal point is not written.

$$\begin{array}{r} 0.46875 \\ 32\overline{\smash{)}15.00000} \\ \underline{128} \\ 220 \\ \underline{192} \\ 280 \\ \underline{256} \\ 240 \\ \underline{224} \\ 160 \\ \underline{160} \\ 0 \end{array}$$

The quotient is 0.46875.

Rounding Decimal Numbers

In the hospital situation, decimals beyond hundredths are seldom used since the measuring devices for administering dosages are not sensitive enough to give accuracy beyond hundredths. Few instruments the nurse uses are accurate beyond hundredths.

When a computation involves division, the decimal results should be rounded off. To round off a decimal to the nearest tenths, consider the numeral in the hundredths position. If the numeral is:

Greater than 5, increase the tenths numeral by 1.

Less than 5, do not increase the tenths numeral.

Equal to 5, increase the tenths numeral if it is odd; do not increase the tenths numeral if it is even.

To round off 0.47 to the nearest tenths, check the value in the hundredths column (7). Since 7 is greater than 5, round the tenths position up and obtain 0.5. Notice that we increase the tenths position to 5 and drop the remaining digits to the right.

Round off 1.329421 to the nearest hundredth.

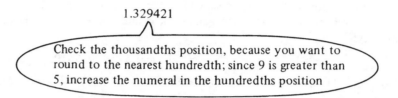

Rounded it is 1.33. Now round the same number to the nearest tenth

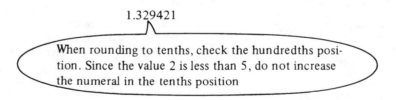

Rounded it is 1.3. Now round off 1.475 to the nearest hundredth.

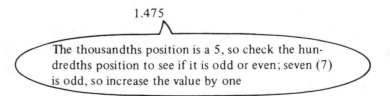

Rounded it is 1.48.

Exercise 7

Change each of the following to decimals. Obtain a second answer by rounding off to the nearest hundredth.

1. $\frac{3}{4}$ 2. $\frac{7}{16}$

3. $\frac{1}{2}$ 4. $\frac{23}{100}$

5. $\frac{7}{8}$ 6. $\frac{1}{20}$

7. $\frac{3}{5}$ 8. $\frac{7}{27}$

9. $\frac{5}{64}$ 10. $\frac{21}{32}$

Decimals to Fractions

To change a decimal to a fraction requires only that one know the positions to the right of the decimal point. To change 0.65 to a fraction, reason that since 0.65 represents 65 hundredths, the fraction would be

$$0.65 = \frac{65}{100}$$

Then reducing to lowest terms gives

$$\frac{65}{100} = \frac{5 \times 13}{5 \times 20} = \frac{13}{20}$$

The fraction representing 0.65 is $\frac{13}{20}$. This fraction is in lowest terms.

Represent 0.751 as a fraction.

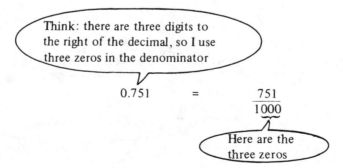

Think: there are three digits to the right of the decimal, so I use three zeros in the denominator

$$0.751 \qquad = \qquad \frac{751}{1000}$$

Here are the three zeros

133651

An alternate approach is to think 0.751 was seven hundred fifty-one thousandths, so the fraction was 751 divided by 1000. This fraction is in lowest terms.

As a rule for changing decimals to fractions, the decimal point is dropped and the appropriate denominator is used.

RULE: To convert a decimal number to a fraction, count the number of digits from the last nonzero digit back to the decimal. Then place the number (without the decimal) in the numerator of the fraction and a 1 with as many zeros as counted under the above reasoning. This yields the fraction equivalent of the decimal number.

EXAMPLE 1.12

Change 0.83141 to a fraction.

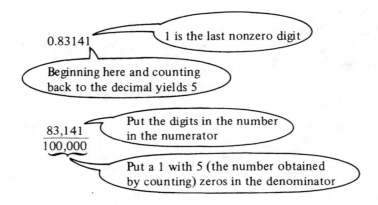

Change 0.615007 to a fraction.

so

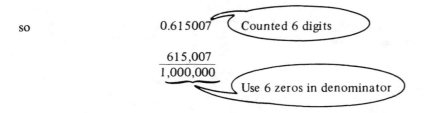

Exercise 8

Change the decimals to fractions:

1. 0.125   2. 0.4

3. 0.921   4. 2.84

5. 0.25   6. 0.02

7. 0.10   8. 0.375

9. 0.75   10. 0.65

Adding and Subtracting Decimals

The addition of decimal numbers is an extension of addition of whole numbers. In adding whole numbers, the units, tens, and hundreds columns are lined up before adding:

$$
\begin{array}{r}
11 \\
43 \\
+625 \\
\hline
679
\end{array}
$$

In order to add decimal numbers the decimal points are lined up vertically so that tenths are added to tenths, hundredths to hundredths, etc.

The usual procedure is to express a number less than 1 so that a zero precedes the decimal point. For instance, the number 91 hundredths is written as 0.91 instead of .91. This practice makes it easier to determine a number with the decimal point inserted in the wrong place by merely noticing that the decimal point is not preceded by a zero. Likewise, zeros may be added following the decimal number without changing the value of the number. This may be useful when adding numbers like 1.37 and 0.1. The method is

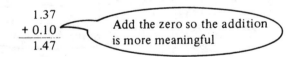

$$
\begin{array}{r}
1.37 \\
+0.10 \\
\hline
1.47
\end{array}
$$

Add the zero so the addition is more meaningful

For example, add 0.94, 1.35, and 0.813:

$$
\begin{array}{r}
0.940 \\
1.350 \\
+0.813 \\
\hline
3.103
\end{array}
$$

When subtracting decimal numbers, the same general procedure is used in that the decimal numbers are aligned vertically so that the decimal points are exactly underneath each other. For example, subtract 0.735 from 1.869

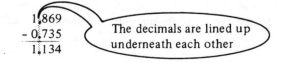

$$
\begin{array}{r}
1.869 \\
-0.735 \\
\hline
1.134
\end{array}
$$

The decimals are lined up underneath each other

Exercise 9

Add or subtract the decimals using the indicated operation:

1. $1.394 + 2.877$

2. $0.716 + 1.82$

3. $3.52 - 1.91$

4. $7.78 - 1.362$

5. $11.1 + 0.37$

6. $19.3 + 5 + 10.07$

7. $8.1 - 1.22 - 0.56$

8. $522.7 - 16.941$

9. $2 - 0.0065$

10. $1.25 - 1.0025$

Multiplying Decimals

When multiplying decimal numbers, most of the ordinary principles of multiplying numbers are unchanged. The numbers are lined up with the right-hand digits under each other. For example, for 514.3 times 2.13 write

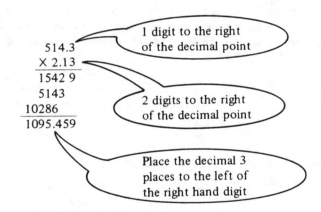

The digits are multiplied in the usual manner and added in the columns.

The difference in the usual procedure occurs when the decimal point is to be placed in the result to obtain the final answer. To place the decimal correctly, first count the number of digits to the right of the decimal point in each of the two numbers being multiplied together. The sum of these two numbers of digits to the right of the decimal points is the number of digits that should appear to the right of the decimal point in the final answer. Second, place the decimal point in the appropriate place.

EXAMPLE 1.13

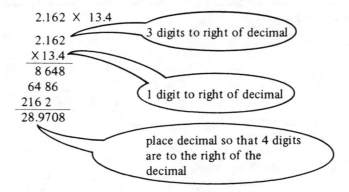

Exercise 10

1. 1.25 × 3.1

2. 0.0013 × 7.6

3. 5.05 × 1.6

4. 2.5 × 2

5. 0.75 × 82.5

6. 5 × 0.719

7. 3.002 × 55

8. 0.95 × 0.02

9. 0.05 × 0.25

10. 40 × 0.35

Dividing Decimals

Figure 1-2 shows the names of the particular components of a division problem.

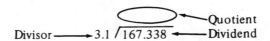

Figure 1-2

Before beginning the actual division, one should place the decimal point in the quotient position. This is accomplished by moving the decimal in the divisor to the right to make it a whole number. Then move the decimal point in the dividend to the right the same number of places. The decimal point in the quotient belongs directly above the decimal position in the dividend. A mnemonic device is provided in Figure 1-3.

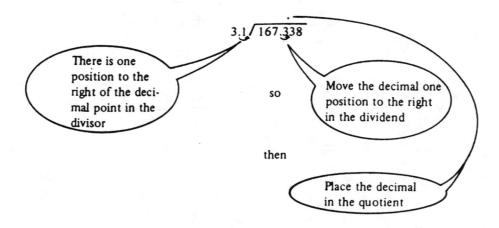

Figure 1-3

Once the decimal is placed in the quotient, the decimal is disregarded throughout the remainder of the division. The usual rules of longhand division are used to find the digits in the quotient. The example below completes the division of the problem in Figures 1-2 and 1-3.

EXAMPLE 1.14

$$
\begin{array}{r}
53.98 \\
3.1\overline{)167.338} \quad \textit{Answer 53.98} \\
\underline{155} \\
123 \\
\underline{93} \\
303 \\
\underline{279} \\
248 \\
\underline{248}
\end{array}
$$

Exercise 11

Divide the following numbers:

1. $9 \div 6$

2. $12.3 \div 3$

3. $192 \div 0.3$

4. $1.92 \div 0.3$

5. $17.651 \div 0.02$

6. $1.0084 \div 0.25$

7. $0.085 \div 0.5$

8. $84 \div 0.035$

9. $18.615 \div 2$

10. $100 \div 0.08$

Percent

Percent means parts in a hundred, so 49 percent means $\frac{49}{100}$, 71 percent means $\frac{71}{100}$, and 15 percent means $\frac{15}{100}$. Since 49 percent means $\frac{49}{100}$, which equals 0.49, a percent may be expressed as a decimal.

RULE: To change a percent to a decimal, drop the percent sign and move the decimal two places to the left.

EXAMPLE 1.15

Chance each percent to a decimal:

$$47\% = 0.47$$
$$18.3\% = 0.183$$
$$14.97\% =$$
$$23\% =$$
$$2\% =$$

Any decimal number can be expressed as parts in 100, thus as a percent. Consider $0.33 = \frac{33}{100}$. Thus 0.33 is the same as 33 percent. The decimal number

$$0.125 = \frac{125}{1000} = \frac{12.5}{100}$$

which is the same as 12.5 percent.

RULE: When changing a decimal to a percent, move the decimal point two places to the right and add the percent sign.

EXAMPLE 1.16

Write the following decimals as percents:

$$0.18 = 18.\% = 18\%$$
$$0.734 =$$
$$0.1257 =$$
$$0.08 =$$
$$0.076 =$$
$$0.10 =$$

Exercise 12

Change the percents to decimals:

1. 4%   **2.** 18%

3. 0.5%   **4.** 85%

5. 63.4%

Change the decimals to percents:

6. 0.94   **7.** 0.02

8. 0.007   **9.** 0.845

10. 0.034

RATIO AND PROPORTIONS

Ratios

Two quantities are often expressed in terms of their relationship to each other. The expression

4 pencils for 10 cents

indicates that

	Relationship
4 cost 10 cents	4 to 10
8 cost 20 cents	8 to 20
12 cost 30 cents	12 to 30

Thus there is a fixed relationship between the number of pencils and their cost. When the number of pencils is compared with the cost, a ratio is used.

A *ratio* is a comparison between two quantities. Ratios are most frequently associated with fractional numbers. The two terms of the ratio become the numerator and denominator of the fraction.

Another notation that is often used is

$$a \text{ to } b \quad \text{or} \quad \frac{a}{b} \quad \text{or} \quad a:b$$

The statement "4 pencils for 10 cents" means the ratio of pencils to cents is 4 to 10. This may be expressed

$$4 \text{ to } 10 \quad \text{or} \quad \frac{4}{10} \quad \text{or} \quad 4:10$$

The fraction form (or quotient form) of expressing ratios will be stressed here because it allows the easiest solution to problems.

The ratio of triangles to circles

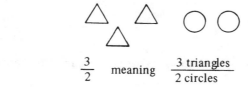

is 3 to 2, $\qquad \frac{3}{2}$ meaning $\frac{3 \text{ triangles}}{2 \text{ circles}}$

The comparison in this case is triangles to circles.

Ratios are often given as a rate. Consider

$$3 \text{ inches per hour}$$

The ratio is

$$3 \text{ inches to } 1 \text{ hour} \quad \frac{3 \text{ inches}}{1 \text{ hour}}$$

The phrase "per hour" implies "per *one* hour." Expressions of this sort are often written 3 in/h, where the diagonal or slash bar is read "per."

EXAMPLE 1.17

A nursing school has 28 male students and 76 female students. What is the ratio of male students to female students?

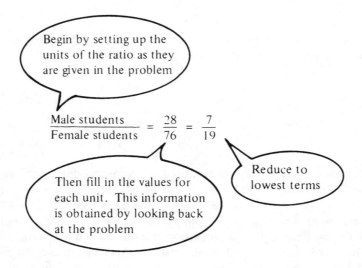

Exercise 13

Solve the following:

1. For every 7 nurses in Winnfield, there are 2 doctors.
  a. What is the ratio of doctors to nurses?
  b. What is the ratio of nurses to doctors?

2. A player hits 8 baskets in 11 shots. What is the ratio of baskets to shots?

3. Of the 57 nursing students, 19 are male. What is the ratio of female students to male students?

4. A metal is packaged so that there are 3 ounces of gold per 15 ounces of metal. What is the ratio of gold to metal?

5. In a coal mine, 36 people load each conveyor belt. Each belt carries 18 cubic feet of coal per minute. What is the ratio of cubic feet of coal per minute?

Proportions

Proportions are the primary method used in computing drug problems. A *proportion* is a statement of equality between two ratios. Often the nurse is faced with a drug order with a dosage that differs from the way the drug is labeled. That is, the desired dosage (the dosage ordered by the physician for the patient) is to contain a certain amount of the drug, but the on-hand drug contains a different amount of the drug. By using proportions the nurse can quickly compute the amount of the available drug (on hand) that is needed to administer the medication ordered by the physician.

The objective in this section is to learn a method for solving proportions. We will develop an algorithm (a set of rules for solving a problem) and learn to use the algorithm.

To begin the development of an algorithm, let us investigate the use of proportion in showing the equality of two fractions. Reread the definition of a proportion. From the work done in previous sections, $\frac{1}{2}$ and $\frac{5}{10}$ are equal fractions; that is, by renaming fractions

$$\frac{1}{2} = \frac{1 \times 5}{2 \times 5} = \frac{5}{10}$$

But proportions can also be used to determine when two fractions are equal.

To show the fractions $\frac{1}{2}$ and $\frac{5}{10}$ are equal, set up a proportion (a statement of equality between ratios or fractions):

$$\frac{1}{2} \overset{?}{=} \frac{5}{10}$$

If the two fractions are equal, then

$$1 \times 10 \overset{?}{=} 2 \times 5$$
$$10 = 10$$

Yes, the fractions are equal. Notice where the numbers in the product were located in the proportion. This has often been called a *cross product,*

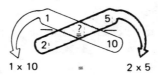

$$1 \times 10 \qquad = \qquad 2 \times 5$$

meaning the numerator of one fraction (1) multiplied by the denominator of the second fraction (10) is equal to the denominator of the first fraction (2) multiplied by the numerator of the second fraction (5). Notice the X or cross pattern to the multiplication. Four-eights is the same as five-tenths. Using proportion to verify this fact, set the fractions equal

$$\frac{4}{8} = \frac{5}{10}$$

Cross-multiplying gives

$$4 \times 10 = 5 \times 8$$
$$40 = 40$$

Since both terms in the cross product equal 40, the fractions are equal.

Consider two fractions known to be unequal, such as one-half and three-fourths. Use proportions to show one-half does not equal three-fourths.

$$\frac{1}{2} \overset{?}{=} \frac{3}{4}$$
$$1 \times 4 \overset{?}{=} 2 \times 3$$
$$4 \overset{?}{=} 6 \quad \text{No!}$$

Since 4 does not equal 6, the original fractions were not equal.

EXAMPLE 1.18

Use proportions to investigate the equality of the following fractions:

$\frac{1}{8}, \frac{5}{40}$ $\frac{1}{8} \overset{?}{=} \frac{5}{40}$ $1 \times 40 \overset{?}{=} 5 \times 8$ $40 = 40$ Equal

$\frac{3}{7}, \frac{6}{14}$ $\frac{3}{\Box} \overset{?}{=} \frac{\Box}{\Box}$ $\Box \times 14 \overset{?}{=} \Box \times \Box$ $\Box \overset{?}{=} \Box$ _____

$\frac{7}{8}, \frac{21}{24}$ $\frac{\Box}{\Box} \overset{?}{=} \frac{\Box}{\Box}$ $\Box \times \Box \overset{?}{=} \Box \times \Box$ $\Box \overset{?}{=} \Box$ _____

$\frac{3}{4}, \frac{9}{11}$ $\frac{\Box}{\Box} \overset{?}{=} \frac{\Box}{\Box}$ $\Box \times 11 \overset{?}{=} \Box \times 9$ $\Box \overset{?}{=} \Box$ _____

Let us extend the idea of a proportion as the statement of equality between ratios (two fractions). Consider the case where one ratio is given and the second has an undetermined component. For instance, suppose you are given the proportion

$$\frac{1}{2} = \frac{n}{10}$$

where the value of n is to be determined so that a true statement results. Using the above examples as a guide,

$$\frac{1}{2} = \frac{n}{10}$$

means

$$2 \times n = 1 \times 10$$

which yields the equation

$$2n = 10$$

Note that $2 \times n$ is the same as $2n$ meaning two times n. Also when we see n, we will know that means $1 \times n$.

In order to solve this equation, use the following logic

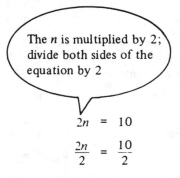

The n is multiplied by 2; divide both sides of the equation by 2

$$2n = 10$$

$$\frac{2n}{2} = \frac{10}{2}$$

but with $\frac{2n}{2}$ we can cancel and obtain n.

$$\frac{\cancel{2}n}{\cancel{2}} = \frac{10}{2}$$

$$n = \frac{10}{2} = 5$$

The result is 5; that is, the value of n which makes the proportion a true statement is 5. Solve the following example.

EXAMPLE 1.19

$$\frac{3}{4} = \frac{n}{36}$$

Cross-multiplying gives $\boxed{} \times n = 3 \times \boxed{}$

Cancel $\dfrac{\boxed{} \times n}{\boxed{}} = \dfrac{3 \times \boxed{}}{\boxed{}}$

$$n = \frac{3 \times \boxed{}}{\boxed{}}$$

$$n = \boxed{}$$

Solving another problem:

$$\frac{1}{8} = \frac{n}{32}$$

$$8n = 32(1) \qquad 8\overline{)32.}^{\,4}$$

$$n = \frac{32}{8} \qquad \frac{32}{0}$$

$$n = 4$$

Consider the following problem:

> Two pints of honey fill five cups. How many pints of honey will it take to fill 14 cups?

First, set up the ratio given in the first sentence:

$$\frac{2 \text{ pints}}{5 \text{ cups}}$$

Now use the second sentence to set up a ratio using the same units:

$$\frac{? \text{ pints}}{14 \text{ cups}}$$

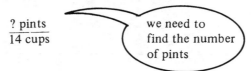
we need to find the number of pints

Let x = the number of pints and set the ratios equal:

$$\frac{2}{5} = \frac{x}{14}$$

cross multiplying

$$5x = (2)(14)$$

$$5x = 28$$

$$x = \frac{28}{5} = 5.6$$

5.6 cups of honey are needed.

EXAMPLE 1.20

A medicine contains 5 grams in two tablets. How many grams are in six tablets?

1. What is the ratio of grams to tablets in the first sentence?

2. Set up a ratio of grams to tablets using the second sentence (use x to represent the number of grams).

3. Set up a proportion using the two ratios.

4. Solve the proportion to find the number of grams.

Exercise 14

Solve the following proportions:

1. $\frac{2}{3} = \frac{x}{15}$

2. $\frac{x}{12} = \frac{3}{4}$

3. $\frac{x}{1.08} = \frac{4}{5}$

4. $\frac{17}{25} = \frac{x}{1000}$

5. $\frac{x}{250} = \frac{12}{30}$

6. $\frac{175}{1} = \frac{x}{500}$

7. $\frac{x}{\frac{1}{2}} = \frac{10}{1}$

8. $\frac{1}{\frac{1}{100}} = \frac{x}{4}$

9. $\frac{5}{100} = \frac{x}{320}$

10. $\frac{16}{80} = \frac{x}{5}$

Solve using proportions:

11. If a car can travel 81 miles on 6 gallons of gasoline, how far can it go on 22 gallons?

12. If the juice of two oranges fills three-fifths of a cup, then how many oranges does it take to fill 3 cups?

13. How many eggs does it take to weigh 5 pounds if 14 eggs weigh $2\frac{1}{3}$ pounds?

14. Two boys divide 32 marbles in the ratio of 5 to 3. How many marbles does each boy get? (Hint: each boy gets what part of the total?)

15. A medicine has 2 grams in every three tablets. How many grams are in five tablets?

16. A mixture contains 3 quarts of alcohol in 8 quarts of solution. How much alcohol is in 20 quarts of solution?

17. A syrup recipe calls for 4 pounds of sugar for 7 pounds of berries. How many pounds of sugar are needed for 10 pounds of berries?

18. In problem 17, how many pounds of berries would be needed for 5 pounds of sugar?

Posttest

This test will serve as an arithmetic assessment of the topics covered in this chapter. Express the Hindu-Arabic numerals as Roman numerals:

1. 12   = _____   2. 5   = _____

3. 20   = _____   4. 19   = _____

5. 2   = _____   6. 6   = _____

Express the Roman numerals as Hindu-Arabic numerals:

7. xv   = _____   8. iv   = _____

9. XLIII = _____   10. viii   = _____

11. XXX   = _____   12. VII   = _____

13. For the fraction $\frac{19}{32}$, 32 is the _____

Are the fractions equal (yes or no)?

14. $\frac{2}{3}, \frac{12}{18}$ **15.** $\frac{4}{7}, \frac{16}{28}$

Reduce the fractions to lowest terms:

16. $\frac{9}{48}$ **17.** $\frac{25}{50}$

18. $\frac{14}{21}$ **19.** $\frac{14}{39}$

Change the mixed numbers to fractions:

20. $2\frac{1}{3}$ **21.** $11\frac{3}{10}$

22. $21\frac{4}{5}$

Perform the indicated operation (express answers in the simplest form):

23. $\frac{5}{7} \times \frac{3}{4}$ = _____   **24.** $\frac{2}{3} \times \frac{5}{8}$ = _____

25. $2\frac{1}{2} \times \frac{2}{5}$ = _____   **26.** $\frac{3}{8} \div \frac{2}{3}$ = _____

27. $\frac{4}{5} \div 3$ = _____   **28.** $17 \div 8$ = _____

29. $\dfrac{\frac{2}{3}}{\frac{5}{8}}$ = _____   **30.** $1 \div \frac{1}{4}$ = _____

31. $5\overline{)4}$ = _____   **32.** $1.37 + 2.84$ = _____

33. $6.45 - 3.87$ = _____   **34.** 3.14×2.2 = _____

35. 0.017×1.36 = _____   **36.** $7.21 \div 0.5$ = _____

37. $0.0314 \div 0.14$ = _____

Change the percents to decimals:

38. 5% = _____

39. 0.7% = _____

40. 37% = _____

41. 1.2% = _____

Change the decimals to percents:

42. 0.45 = _____

43. 0.02   = _____

44. 0.187 = _____

45. 0.0125 = _____

Solve the following for the value of x:

46. $\dfrac{3}{7} = \dfrac{x}{21}$

47. $\dfrac{3}{11} = \dfrac{x}{7}$

48. $\dfrac{x}{10} = \dfrac{4}{5}$

49. $\dfrac{1}{300} = \dfrac{x}{450}$

50. $\dfrac{1}{100} = \dfrac{x}{1000}$

51. $\dfrac{1}{50} = \dfrac{x}{50}$

ANSWERS TO EXAMPLES

Example 1.3

5 plus 3, or 8
10 plus 2, or 12
25
30 plus 5 plus 2, or 37

Example 1.4

500 minus 100, or 400
10 minus 1, or 9
100 minus 10, or 90
5 minus 1, or 4

Example 1.6

5, 7, 4, 5

Example 1.7

$$\frac{15}{50} = \frac{3 \times 5}{10 \times 5} = \frac{3}{10}$$

$$\frac{21}{35} = \frac{3 \times 7}{5 \times 7} = \frac{3}{5}$$

$$\frac{54}{66} = \frac{9 \times 6}{11 \times 6} = \frac{9}{11}$$

$$\frac{32}{80} = \frac{2 \times 16}{5 \times 16} = \frac{2}{5}$$

$$\frac{28}{64} = \frac{7 \times 4}{16 \times 4} = \frac{7}{16}$$

$$\frac{8}{32} = \frac{1 \times 8}{4 \times 8} = \frac{1}{4}$$

Example 1.8

$$5\frac{3}{8} = \frac{5 \times 8 + 3}{8} = \frac{40 + 3}{8} = \frac{43}{8}$$

$$3\frac{5}{11} = \frac{3 \times 11 + 5}{11} = \frac{33 + 5}{11} = \frac{38}{11}$$

$$2\frac{7}{9} = \frac{2 \times 9 + 7}{9} = \frac{18 + 7}{9} = \frac{25}{9}$$

Example 1.9

1. 30; least multiple of 5 and 6 is 5 times 6.

2. $\frac{2}{5} = \frac{12}{30}$

3. $\frac{1}{6} = \frac{5}{30}$

4. $\frac{2}{5} + \frac{1}{6} = \frac{12}{30} + \frac{5}{30} = \frac{12 + 5}{30} = \frac{17}{30}$

Example 1.15

14.97% = 0.1497
23% = 0.23
2% = 0.02

Example 1.16

0.734 = 73.4%
0.1257 = 12.57%
0.08 = 8%
0.076 = 7.6%
0.10 = 10%

Example 1.18

$\dfrac{3}{7} \overset{?}{=} \dfrac{6}{14}$ $3 \times 14 \overset{?}{=} 7 \times 6$ $42 \overset{?}{=} 42$ Equal

$\dfrac{7}{8} \overset{?}{=} \dfrac{21}{24}$ $7 \times 24 \overset{?}{=} 8 \times 21$ $168 \overset{?}{=} 168$ Equal

$\dfrac{3}{4} \overset{?}{=} \dfrac{9}{11}$ $3 \times 11 \overset{?}{=} 4 \times 9$ $33 \overset{?}{=} 36$ Unequal

Example 1.19

$$4 \times n = 3 \times 36$$

$$\frac{4 \times n}{4} = \frac{3 \times 36}{4}$$

$$n = \frac{3 \times 36}{4}$$

$$n = 27$$

Example 1.20

1. $\dfrac{5 \text{ grams}}{2 \text{ tablets}}$

2. $\dfrac{x \text{ grams}}{6 \text{ tablets}}$

3. $\dfrac{5}{2} = \dfrac{x}{6}$

4. $\dfrac{5}{2} = \dfrac{x}{6}$
   $2x = (5)(6)$
   $2x = 30$
   $x = \dfrac{30}{2} = 15$

2 SYSTEMS OF MEASUREMENT

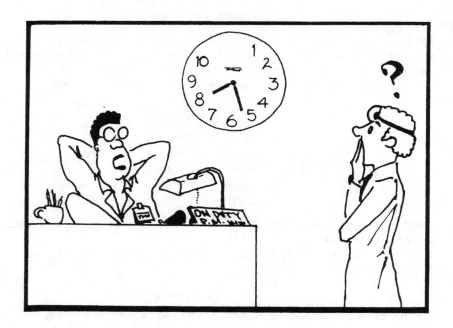

Metric conversion, doctor . . . shortened the night shift by two hours!

CHAPTER OBJECTIVES

- Perform calculations in the metric system of measure
- Convert units of measure within the metric, apothecaries', and household systems of measure
- Demonstrate proficiency with symbols in the metric, apothecaries', and household systems of measure
- Utilize the proportion method when changing units of measure from one system to another

INTRODUCTION

The two basic systems of weight and measure in the United States are the metric system and the apothecaries' system. There is a definite trend toward adoption of the metric system exclusively, but since both systems are currently in use, nurses must be familiar with both and be able to use them interchangeably.

A third system of measure the nurse often needs is the household system of measure. This is the least accurate system of measure and is used only when it is not feasible to calculate and measure dosage by the metric or apothecaries' system. The household system of measure is generally used by nurses and patients in the home. Such familiar household measures as the teaspoon, tablespoon, ounce, drop, and glassful may be substituted for approximate equivalents of the two major systems of measure.

THE METRIC SYSTEM

The metric system was devised by the French in 1791 in an effort to simplify measurement. The metric system is based on a uniform decimal system (a system of multiples or powers of 10).

The metric system utilizes three units of measure with which the nurse needs to be familiar:

$$\text{Liter (l)} = \text{unit of volume}$$
$$\text{Gram (g)} = \text{unit of weight}$$
$$\text{Meter (m)} = \text{unit of length}$$

The abbreviations for each of the units is the first letter of each word, so for the gram the abbreviation is g. The abbreviations L., Gm., and M. for liters, grams, and meters, respectively, were formerly used in medical texts and may still be found in other sources.

To express multiples and parts of units, six basic prefixes are used:

Prefix			Symbol
kilo	=	1000 units	k
hecto	=	100 units	h
deka	=	10 units	da
deci	=	0.1 unit	d
centi	=	0.01 unit	c
milli	=	0.001 unit	m

Note that the abbreviation for each prefix is its first letter except for deka (da), where two letters are needed to distinguish between deka (da) and deci (d).

When a measurement is expressed in the metric system, a prefix and unit may be used. An example of a metric measurement is

47 milligrams

Two pieces of information are contained in the word milligram. First, the prefix, *milli-*, indicates the measure is in thousandths of a unit. Second, the unit indicates whether length, weight, or volume has been measured. In this case, the unit is gram, so the measurement is a weight measure. Thus, 47 milligrams means 47 thousandths of a gram, that is, 47 thousandths of a unit of weight. The abbreviation for 47 milligrams is

47 mg

When a prefix is written with the unit of measure, the abbreviation for the prefix is followed by the abbreviation for the unit.

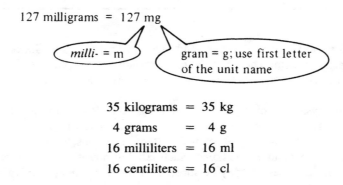

$$127 \text{ milligrams} = 127 \text{ mg}$$

milli- = m

gram = g; use first letter of the unit name

$$35 \text{ kilograms} = 35 \text{ kg}$$
$$4 \text{ grams} = 4 \text{ g}$$
$$16 \text{ milliliters} = 16 \text{ ml}$$
$$16 \text{ centiliters} = 16 \text{ cl}$$

EXAMPLE 2.1*

Along with the numerical data, provide the abbreviation if the name is given or the name if the abbreviation is given.

18 milliliters = _____ ml

4 cl = _____ centiliters

5 centigrams = 5 _____

7 meters = _____

2 kilograms = _____

3 dl = _____

5 cm = _____

The unit for weight, the *gram,* is equal to the weight of water contained in a 1 centimeter cube and at a temperature of 4°C. The water is at 4° because that is the temperature at which water is densest (and the most water can be contained in the cube).

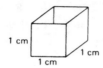

The unit for liquid measure, the *liter,* is the volume of fluid contained in a cube that is 10 centimeters on each edge. The volume of a cube 10 cm by 10 cm by 10 cm is 10 cm × 10 cm × 10 cm, or 1000 cubic centimeters (cm³).

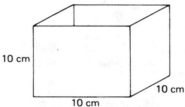

So   1 liter = 1000 cm³ = 1000 cc

Cubic centimeters (cm³) are commonly referred to as cc

Thus, 1 liter is 1000 cm³ (1000 cc). From previous discussions, 1 liter equals 1000 milliliters. Thus

$$1 \text{ liter} = 1000 \text{ cm}^3$$
$$1 \text{ liter} = 1000 \text{ ml}$$
$$1000 \text{ cm}^3 = 1000 \text{ ml}$$
$$1 \text{ cm}^3 = 1 \text{ ml}$$

Although 1 cm³ is the same as 1 ml of fluid, 1 ml is the preferred abbreviation. The older form (1 cc) is still common, however.

---

*Answers to examples appear on pages 72-74.

The nurse usually works with grams or liters. The meter is seldom used. For the liter, the relationships between prefixes and units are

1000 liters	=	1 kiloliter	1 kl	=	1000 liters
100 liters	=	1 hectoliter	1 hl	=	100 liters
10 liters	=	1 dekaliter	1 dal	=	10 liters
1 liter	=	1 liter			
1 liter	=	10 deciliters	1 dl	=	0.1 liter
1 liter	=	100 centiliters	1 cl	=	0.01 liter
1 liter	=	1000 milliliters	1 ml	=	0.001 liter

Likewise, for the gram unit of weight

1 kg	=	1000 g	1 g	=	0.001 kg
1 hg	=	100 g	1 g	=	0.01 hg
1 dag	=	10 g	1 g	=	0.1 dag
1 g	=	1 g			
1 dg	=	0.1 g	1 g	=	10 dg
1 cg	=	0.01 g	1 g	=	100 cg
1 mg	=	0.001 g	1 g	=	1000 mg

Converting Units Within the Metric System

For the nurse, the most frequent conversions involve liters and milliliters or grams and milligrams.

TABLE 2.1
Metric table of weight, volume, and length

Metric weight (dry)

1 gram (g) = 1000 milligrams (mg)	1 mg = 0.001 gm
1000 grams (g) = 1 kilogram (kg)	0.001 kg = 1 g

Metric volume (wet)

1 liter = 1000 milliliters (ml)	1 ml = 0.001 liter
1000 liters = 1 kiloliter (kl)	0.001 kl = 1 liter

Metric length

1 meter (m) = 100 centimeters (cm)	1 cm = 0.01 m
1 meter (m) = 1000 millimeters (mm)	1 mm = 0.001 m
1 centimeter (cm) = 10 millimeters (mm)	1 mm = 0.1 cm
1000 meters (m) = 1 kilometer (km)	1 m = 0.001 km

Two methods for converting in the metric system are presented below, one using ratio and proportion and the second using rules. Although using the rules is simpler than using ratio and proportion when converting in this system, the proportion method will be essential later for solving drug problems successfully. Practicing the proportion method in these simple situations will make it easier in later chapters.

Convert 500 ml to liters. The problem stated mathematically is

$$500 \text{ ml} = \underline{\hspace{1.5cm}} \text{ liters}$$

From the given problem, write a ratio

$$\frac{500 \text{ ml}}{x \text{ liters}}$$

Once the ratio is written, determine an equivalence between the units used in the ratio. Here 1000 ml is the same as 1 liter:

$$1000 \text{ ml} = 1 \text{ liter}$$

Use the values in the equivalence to write another ratio (make sure the units in the numerator and denominator are the same as in the first ratio):

$$\frac{1000 \text{ ml}}{1 \text{ liter}}$$

In both cases the ratio is milliliters to liters. Set the two ratios equal

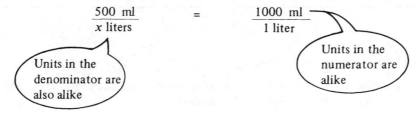

Use the numerical values and the method of cross-multiplying to solve for x:

$$\frac{500}{x} = \frac{1000}{1}$$

$$1000 \, x = 1 \times 500$$

$$1000 \, x = 500$$

$$x = \frac{500}{1000} = \frac{5}{10} = \frac{1}{2} = 0.5$$

$$x = 0.5 \text{ liter}$$

EXAMPLE 2.2

Solve the following:

$$450 \text{ ml} = \underline{\hspace{0.5cm}x\hspace{0.5cm}} \text{ liters}$$

1. Write a ratio from the given problem.

2. Determine an equivalence between the given units.

3. Write a ratio using equivalence in step 2.

4. Set the two ratios equal. (Are like units in the numerators?)

5. Use the numerical values in the proportion to solve for x.

EXAMPLE 2.3

Solve

$$38 \text{ g} = \underline{\hspace{2cm}} \text{ mg}$$

Use the above example as a guide if necessary.

EXAMPLE 2.4

Solve

$$54 \text{ cm} = \underline{\hspace{2cm}} \text{ m}$$

Remember to set up a proportion.

Rules

In each case that follows, a problem is solved using substitution and logic. Then, the rule is stated and is followed by guided application to a few problems.

Consider converting

$$3 \text{ liters} = \underline{\hspace{2cm}} \text{ ml}$$

From the table, each liter equals 1000 ml. Note that 3 liters = 3 (1 liter). Substitute 1000 ml for 1 liter:

$$3 \text{ liters} = 3 (1 \text{ liter}) = 3 (1000 \text{ ml}) = 3000 \text{ ml}$$

Substituting
1 liter = 1000 ml

Recall from Chapter 1 that 3.0 = 3; thus

$$3 \text{ liters} = 3.0 \text{ liters}$$

and from the above work

$$3.0 \text{ liters} = 3000 \text{ ml}$$

RULE 1: *Liters to milliliters* To change liters to milliliters, multiply the number of liters by 1000 or move the decimal point three places to the right.

RULE 2: *Grams to milligrams* To change grams to milligrams, multiply the number of grams by 1000 or move the decimal point three places to the right.

RULE 3: *Meters to millimeters* To change meters to millimeters, multiply the number of meters by 1000 or move the decimal point three places to the right.

EXAMPLE 2.5

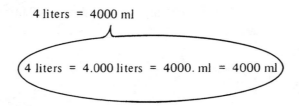

4 liters = 4000 ml

(4 liters = 4.000 liters = 4000. ml = 4000 ml)

6 liters = _____ ml
0.3 liter = _____ ml
7 g = _____ mg
15 m = _____ mm

Now consider changing milliliters to liters. Change

$$600 \text{ ml} = \underline{\hspace{2cm}} \text{ liters}$$

From Table 2.1, 1 ml = 0.001 liter. Note also

$$600 \text{ ml} = 600 \text{ (1 ml)}$$

Substituting gives

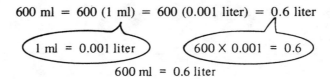

600 ml = 600 (1 ml) = 600 (0.001 liter) = 0.6 liter

(1 ml = 0.001 liter)   (600 × 0.001 = 0.6)

Thus   600 ml = 0.6 liter

RULE 4: *Milliliters to liters* To change milliliters to liters, multiply the number of milliliters by 0.001 or move the decimal point three places to the left.

RULE 5: *Milligrams to grams* To change milligrams to grams, multiply the number of milligrams by 0.001 or move the decimal point three places to the left.

RULE 6: *Millimeters to meters* To change millimeters to meters, multiply the number of millimeters by 0.001 or move the decimal point three places to the left.

EXAMPLE 2.6

Change the following as indicated.

$$480 \text{ ml} = 0.480 \text{ liter}$$

480 ml = 480.0 ml = 0.480 liter

750 ml = _____ liters
9800 mg = _____ g
42 mm = _____ m

RULE 7: *Kiloliters to liters* To change kiloliters to liters, multiply the number of kiloliters by 1000 or move the decimal point three places to the right.

RULE 8: *Kilograms to grams* To change the kilograms to grams, multiply the number of kilograms by 1000 or move the decimal point three places to the right.

RULE 9: *Kilometers to meters* To change kilometers to meters, multiply the number of kilometers by 1000 or move the decimal three places to the right.

EXAMPLE 2.7

Change the kilograms (kilometers) to grams (meters).

$$2.0 \text{ kg} = 2000 \text{ g}$$

2.0 kg = 2 (1 kg) = 2(1000 g) = 2000 g
Thus 2.0 kg = 2 0 0 0. g by rule 8

4 kg = _____ g
4.23 kg = _____ g
0.543 kg = _____ g
2.57 km = _____ m

When changing grams to kilograms, as in the problem

$$349 \text{ g} = \underline{\hspace{2cm}} \text{ kg}$$

recall that 1 g equals 0.001 kg. Also, 349 g = 349 (1 g); then

$$349 \text{ g} = 349(1 \text{ g}) = 349(0.001 \text{ kg}) = 0.349 \text{ kg}$$

1 g = 0.001 kg   349 × 0.001 = 0.349

RULE 10:   *Liters to kiloliters* To change liters to kiloliters, multiply the number of liters by 0.001 or move the decimal point three places to the left.

RULE 11:   *Grams to kilograms* To change grams to kilograms, multiply the number of grams by 0.001 or move the decimal point three places to the left.

RULE 12:   *Meters to kilometers* To change meters to kilometers, multiply the number of meters by 0.001 or move the decimal three places to the left.

EXAMPLE 2.8

Change the grams (liters or meters) to kilograms (kiloliters or kilometers).

1748 g = 1.748 kg

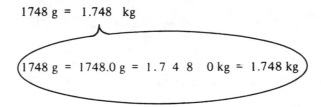

1748 g = 1748.0 g = 1. 7 4 8   0 kg = 1.748 kg

1545 g = _____ kg
45 liters = _____ kl
137 m = _____ km

There are two additional rules necessary to complete metric system measures commonly used in everyday work. These involve the use of centimeters.

RULE 13:   *Meters to centimeters* To change meters to centimeters, multiply the number of meters by 100 or move the decimal point two places to the right.

RULE 14:   *Centimeters to meters* To change centimeters to meters, multiply the number of centimeters by 0.01 or move the decimal point two places to the left.

Exercise 15

Complete the following using rules:

1. 1000 cc = _____ liters

2. 500 liters = _____ ml

3. 60 ml = _____ liters

4. 0.0080 liter = _____ ml

5. 25 mm = _____ m

6. 1 g = _____ mg

7. 250 mg = _____ g

8. 6 g = _____ mg

9. 2000 g   = _____ kg   10. 3 km   = _____ m

11. 2185 cm = _____ m   12. 8.45 kg   = _____ g

13. 30 liters = _____ kl   14. 3 kl   = _____ liters

15. 40 g   = _____ kg   16. 60 mg   = _____ g

17. 7 m   = _____ km   18. 250 cc   = _____ ml

19. 600 kl   = _____ liters 20. 500 mg   = _____ g

21. 1.4 m   = _____ cm   22. 1000 ml   = _____ liters

23. 10 g   = _____ kg   24. 85 cm   = _____ m

25. 8166 m   = _____ mm   26. 1.02 kg   = _____ g

THE APOTHECARIES' SYSTEM

Although the metric system will inevitably replace the apothecaries' system, the apothecaries' system is still used today by physicians and nurses and will continue to be used for the next few decades. Therefore the nurse must understand both the apothecaries' and the metric systems.

In the apothecaries' system the basic unit for weight is the grain. When the system was established, the dry weight unit, the *grain,* was the weight of a grain of wheat. The abbreviation for grain is gr.

After the grain, the next larger unit of weight in the apothecaries' system is the scruple, but now it is seldom used as a unit. A *scruple* is 20 grains.

The dram is the next larger unit after the scruple. A *dram* is 60 grains. The symbol for the dram, ʒ, can be thought of as a z with a tail. After the dram, the ounce is the next larger unit in the apothecaries' system. An *ounce* equals 8 drams. The symbol for ounce is ℥. Thus

$$1 ℥ = 8 ʒ$$

TABLE 2.2
Apothecaries' weights and measures

Weight (dry)
1 dram (ʒ) = 60 grains (gr)
1 ounce (ʒ) = 8 drams (ʒ)
1 pound (lb) = 12 ounces (ʒ)

Weight (liquid)
1 fluidram (fʒ) = 60 minims (♏)
1 fluidounce (fʒ) = 8 fluidrams (fʒ)
1 pint (pt) = 16 fluidounces (fʒ)
1 quart (qt) = 2 pints (pt)
1 gallon (C) = 4 quarts (qt)

Derived measures
1 ounce (ʒ) = 480 grains (gr)
1 fluidounce (fʒ) = 480 minims (♏)
1 minim (♏) = 1 grain (gr)

(This symbol, ʒ, can be thought of as a "greater than" symbol, $>$, attached to the symbol for dram.) The larger unit is the pound (lb), which equals 12 ounces.

In the apothecaries' system both Roman numerals and Hindu-Arabic numerals are used in writing measurements. When the name is spelled out, Hindu-Arabic numerals are used to express the number value:

$$3 \text{ drams}$$

When the symbol (abbreviation) for the unit is used, Roman numerals may be used to express the number value:

$$ʒiii$$

When Roman numerals are used, they always follow the unit symbol. As discussed in Chapter 1, lowercase letters (i, v, x) are used in writing numbers in the apothecaries' system.

Therefore,

$$1 \text{ ounce} = 8 \text{ drams}$$

can be written

$$ʒi = ʒviii$$

Frequently large numbers (50 and over) are expressed using Hindu-Arabic numerals. Fractions are always written using Hindu-Arabic numerals, for example gr $\frac{1}{8}$, gr $\frac{1}{4}$, gr $\frac{1}{16}$. This means that decimals are expressed in fraction form. Decimals should not be used when expressing answers in this system. The fraction $\frac{1}{2}$ occurs so often that a special symbol is used. The Latin word for one-half is *semis,* abbreviated ss

$$7\frac{1}{2} \text{ grains} = \text{gr viiss}$$

EXAMPLE 2.9

What does each abbreviation mean?

1. gr vii = 7 grains
2. ʒ ix = _____
3. ℥ v = _____
4. gr iss = _____
5. gr $\frac{1}{4}$ = _____

The *minim* (♏) is the unit of volume in the apothecaries' system. A minim was defined as the quantity of water weighing the same as one grain of wheat.

In the apothecaries' system the next largest unit of volume is the *fluidram* (fʒ): 1 fluidram is 60 minims.

$$1 \text{ fluidram} = 60 \text{ minims} \quad \text{or} \quad fʒi = 60♏$$

After the fluidram, the next largest unit is the *fluidounce* (f℥): 1 fluidounce (f℥) equals 8 fluidrams. Thus

$$f℥i = fʒviii$$

A *pint* (pt) is 16 fluidounces. Pint is sometimes abbreviated using O, but since this is easily mistaken for zero, the abbreviation pt will be used instead. Two pints equal one *quart* (qt), and four quarts equal one *gallon* (C).

EXAMPLE 2.10

What does each abbreviation mean?

1. fʒ viiss   = _____
2. pt ss   = _____
3. f℥ iv   = _____
4. C iii   = _____
5. ♏ v   = _____

Often it is necessary to change units within the apothecaries' system. Two methods for changing units follow. You should familiarize yourself with both.

Convert 1.5 fluidrams to minims. Mathematically the problem is

$$fʒ \text{ iss} = ♏ \underline{\ \ x\ \ }$$

From the given problem, write a ratio using the given information:

$$\frac{x \text{ minims}}{1.5 \text{ fluidrams}}$$

Once a ratio is written, determine an equivalence between the units used in the ratio (in this case minims and fluidrams).

$$1 \text{ fluidram } = 60 \text{ minims}$$
$$f\!\!\!\;3\,i \; = \; \text{m}60$$

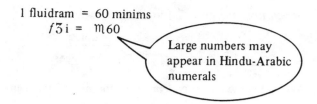

Large numbers may appear in Hindu-Arabic numerals

Form a ratio using the above equivalence; take care to form the second ratio with the same units in numerator and denominator as in the first ratio.

$$\frac{60 \text{ minims}}{1 \text{ fluidram}}$$

The proportion formed from the ratios is

$$\frac{x \text{ minims}}{1.5 \text{ fluidrams}} = \frac{60 \text{ minims}}{1 \text{ fluidram}}$$

In each case the relation is minims to fluidrams. Use the numerical values to solve for x:

$$\frac{x}{1.5} = \frac{60}{1}$$
$$1x = 1.5\,(60)$$
$$x = 90$$

$$\begin{array}{r} 1.5 \\ \times\,60 \\ \hline 90.0 \end{array}$$

Therefore 1.5 fluidrams equals 90 minims.

EXAMPLE 2.11

Convert 2 fluidrams to fluidounces.

$$f\!\!\!\;3\,\text{ii} \; = \; \underline{\hspace{1.5cm}} \; f\!\!\!\;\mathit{3}$$

1. From the given information, complete the ratio

$$\frac{\boxed{} \; f\!\!\!\;\mathit{3}}{\boxed{} \; f\!\!\!\;3}$$

2. Determine an equivalence between fluidrams and fluidounces. *Hint:* Use Table 2.2

3. Write a second ratio from the information in step 2.

4. Set the two ratios equal.

5. Solve for x.

Sometimes the equivalence needed for converting units cannot be obtained directly from Table 2.2. Consider the problem

$$f\!\!\!\;\mathit{3}\,\text{iiss} \; = \; \underline{\hspace{1.5cm}} \; \text{m}$$

The ratio formed from the given information is

$$\frac{x \quad \text{minims}}{2\frac{1}{2} \text{ fluidounces}}$$

Table 2.2 does not show an equivalence for minims and fluidounces, but

$$1 \text{ fluidounce } = 8 \text{ fluidrams}$$

and

$$1 \text{ fluidram } = 60 \text{ minims}$$

These two equivalences can be used to obtain a new equivalence.

$$1 \text{ fluidounce } = 8 \text{ fluidrams } = 8 \, (60 \text{ minims})$$

Each fluidram is 60 minims

So   1 fluidounce = 480 minims

Now a ratio can be formed from the equivalence:

$$\frac{480 \quad \text{minims}}{1 \quad \text{fluidounce}}$$

The proportion formed from the two ratios is

$$\frac{x \quad \text{minims}}{2\frac{1}{2} \text{ fluidounces}} = \frac{480 \quad \text{minims}}{1 \quad \text{fluidounce}}$$

Using the numerical data to solve for x gives

$$\frac{x}{\frac{5}{2}} = \frac{480}{1}$$

$$2\frac{1}{2} = \frac{5}{2}$$

Cross-multiplying, we have

$$1x = \frac{5}{2}(480)$$

$$x = \frac{5 \times 480}{2} = 1200$$

$$= 1200 \, \text{m}$$

$$\begin{array}{r} 480 \\ \times 5 \\ \hline 2400 \end{array}$$

$$\begin{array}{r} 1200 \\ 2\overline{\smash{)}2400} \\ \underline{2} \\ 04 \\ 4 \end{array}$$

EXAMPLE 2.12

Solve the following

$$\text{qt iii} = \underline{\hspace{2cm}} f\mathfrak{z}$$

1. Write a ratio using the given information

2. Determine an equivalence between quarts and fluidounces. *Hint:* Use equivalence for pints and Table 2.2.

3. Write a second ratio using the equivalence from step 2.

4. Set the two ratios equal.

5. Solve for *x*.

Exercise 16

Use proportions to solve the following:

1. qt v = _____ pt   2. $f\mathfrak{z}$ iiiss = _____ $f\mathfrak{z}$

3. C ii = _____ fluidounces   4. ℳ xlv = _____ fluidrams

Although the proportion method for changing units may be used to solve all changes or conversions of units, the changes needed are most often easiest to work using rules. The following rules are useful when changing units in the apothecaries' system of measure.

The rules involve the term *conversion constant*. A conversion constant is a number (obtained from Table 2.2) that aids in changing units of measure. From the table

$$1 \text{ dram} = 60 \text{ grains}$$

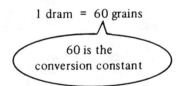

60 is the conversion constant

This equality between the units drams and grains involves a constant, 60. The number 60 is referred to as the conversion constant for drams and grains.

RULE 1: To change from a *larger* unit to a *smaller* unit, multiply the conversion constant by the number value of the larger unit.

RULE 2: To change from a *smaller* unit to a *larger* unit, divide the conversion constant into the number value of the smaller unit.

Consider the problem

$$\mathfrak{z} \text{ iii} = \underline{\hspace{2cm}} \text{gr}$$

The dram unit is larger than the grain unit. Thus the change is from a larger unit to a smaller unit: use Rule 1. From Table 2.2 the conversion constant for drams and grains is 60. Using Rule 1, multiply 60 by the number value of the larger unit (3):

$$60 \times 3 = 180$$

180 grains is equal to 3 drams.

EXAMPLE 2.13

$$\mathfrak{Z} \text{ iss} = \underline{\hspace{2cm}} \mathfrak{Z}$$

1. Rule _____ should be used.
2. What is the conversion constant?
3. How many ounces are given?
4. Find the number of drams.

EXAMPLE 2.14

$$\text{gr cxx} = \underline{\hspace{2cm}} \mathfrak{Z}$$

1. Rule _____ should be used.
2. What is the conversion constant?
3. How many grains are given?
4. Find the number of drams.

Exercise 17

Solve using proportions:

1. gr lxx   = _____ ℨ
2. ℥ xiv   = _____ gr
3. 3 pt   = _____ f℥
4. ℥ xlv   = _____ gr

Solve using one of the rules:

5. 6 qt   = _____ gallons
6. f℥ iiss = _____ ℥
7. ℥ viiss = _____ f℥
8. f℥ xl   = _____ pt
9. 600 gr = _____ ℥
10. ℥ iss   = _____ ℨ
11. ℨ iii   = _____ ℥
12. 7 pt   = _____ f℥

THE HOUSEHOLD SYSTEM

The household system is the least accurate of the three systems of measure. However, these measures may be the only ones the patient is familiar with and may be safely used by the patient who is administering medications at home. The nurse should avoid these measures whenever possible because they are not as accurate as metric and apothecary measures.

TABLE 2.3

Household measures

1 teaspoonful (t) = 60 drops (gtt)
1 tablespoonful (T) = 3 teaspoonsful
1 ounce (oz) = 2 tablespoonsful
1 teacupful = 6 ounces
1 glassful = 8 ounces
1 ounce (oz) = 6 teaspoonsful

The basic unit in the household system is the drop (gtt). The above table contains the equivalent measures in the household system. Many of the names are those commonly used in households today. The ounces referred to above are fluidounces, but the word fluid is generally omitted.

Two methods for changing unit measures are presented. It is suggested that you work with both and adopt the method that is easier for you to understand.

To change units of measure within the household system use ratio and proportions (discussed in Chapter 1). For example,

$$9 \text{ oz} = \underline{\hspace{2cm}} t$$

First set up a ratio using the information given in the problem:

$$\frac{x \text{ t}}{9 \text{ oz}}$$

From Table 2.3 obtain the equivalence for ounces and teaspoonsful:

$$1 \text{ oz} = 6 \text{ t}$$

Set up a ratio using this equivalence, making sure that the units in the numerator and denominator are the same as in the first ratio:

$$\frac{6 \text{ t}}{1 \text{ oz}}$$

Set the two ratios equal and solve for the value of x:

$$\frac{x \text{ t}}{9 \text{ oz}} = \frac{6 \text{ t}}{1 \text{ oz}}$$

$$\frac{x}{9} = \frac{6}{1}$$

$$1x = 9 \ (6)$$

$$x = 9 \ (6) = 54$$

The answer is 54. There are 54 teaspoonsful in 9 ounces.

EXAMPLE 2.15

Changing ounces to drops.

$$3 \text{ oz} = \underline{\quad x \quad} \text{ gtt}$$

1. Set up the ratio from the given problem.

$$\frac{\boxed{\quad} \text{ oz}}{\boxed{\quad} \text{ gtt}}$$

2. From the table set up a ratio involving ounces and drops.
3. Set the two ratios equal.

4. Solve for the value of x.

If you encounter difficulty in step 4, review ratio and proportions in Chapter 1.

Change drops to ounces:

$$180 \text{ gtt} = \underline{\hspace{2cm}} \text{ oz}$$

First, set up a ratio using information in the given problem:

$$\frac{180 \text{ gtt}}{x \text{ oz}}$$

From Table 2.3

$$1 \text{ oz} = 360 \text{ gtt}$$

$$\frac{360 \text{ gtt}}{1 \text{ oz}}$$

Set the two ratios equal:

$$\frac{180 \text{ gtt}}{x \text{ oz}} = \frac{360 \text{ gtt}}{1 \text{ oz}}$$

(Check to make sure like units appear in the two numerators and two denominators.)
Solve for x:

$$\frac{180}{x} = \frac{360}{1}$$

$$360x = 180(1)$$

$$x = \frac{180}{360} = 0.5$$

Thus

$$180 \text{ gtt} = 0.5 \text{ oz}$$

Exercise 18

Use proportions to change units in the household system:

1. 4 T   = _____ t

2. 14 oz = _____ glassfuls

3. 45 gtt = _____ oz

4. 3 t   = _____ T

Another method for changing (or converting) units is the rule method. The same rules used in changing units in the apothecaries' system are useful in the household system. The rules will be presented again but discussed only briefly since they were explained in detail in the previous section.

RULE 1: To change from a *larger* unit to a *smaller* unit, multiply the conversion constant by the number value of the larger unit.

RULE 2: To change from a *smaller* unit to a *larger* unit, divide the conversion constant into the number value of the smaller unit.

Change 3 t to drops:

$$3 \text{ t} = \underline{\hspace{1.5cm}} \text{ gtt}$$

To change a larger measure (teaspoons) to a smaller measure (drops), apply Rule 1. From Table 2.3

$$1 \text{ t} = 60 \text{ gtt}$$

Thus the conversion constant is 60. Applying Rule 1, multiply the conversion constant (60) by the number value of the larger unit (3):

$$60 \times 3 = 180$$

Therefore, 3 teaspoonsful equal 180 drops.

Exercise 19

Solve by applying the correct rule:

1. 30 gtt = _____ t

2. 8 oz   = _____ glassfuls

3. 2 oz   = _____ t

4. 180 gtt = _____ oz

5. 2 T   = _____ oz

6. 1 T   = _____ oz

7. 40 gtt = _____ t

8. 4 t   = _____ gtt

9. 4 oz   = _____ glassfuls

10. 16 oz = _____ glassfuls

11. 2 T   = _____ t

12. 360 gtt = _____ t

13. 9 t   = _____ T

14. 24 oz = _____ glassfuls

15. $\frac{1}{4}$ t   = _____ gtt

EQUIVALENTS

To change units between systems of measure, the proportions method works well. For changing units between the systems the proportion method is set up the same way as in past sections.

TABLE 2.4
Approximate equivalents

Volume				
Metric		**Apothecaries'**		**Household**[1]
1 ml	=	15 ♏ (or 16 ♏)[2]	=	15 gtt
4 ml	=	1 ʒ (fʒ)	=	60 gtt (1 t)
15 ml	=	4 ʒ (fʒ)	=	1 T
30 ml	=	1 ℥ (f℥)	=	2 T
500 ml	=	1 pt		
1000 ml	=	1 qt		

Weight		
Metric		**Apothecaries'**
60 mg (0.06 g)	=	1 gr
1000 mg (1 g)	=	15 gr
4 g	=	1 ʒ
30 g	=	1 ℥

[1] Household equivalents specified are those frequently used. Use the metric or apothecaries' system when measuring dosages because measurements are more accurate.
[2] 1 ml = 15 minims will be used for computational purposes.

The equivalent for 1 milliliter is either 15 or 16 minims. Quite often the value chosen for use depends on whether the numbers involved in the computations are even or odd. This criterion is not theoretically or scientifically supported.

Because the equivalents are approximate, the answer can vary by as much as 10% and still be considered within safe limits. When the nurse rounds the computed answer to either minims or tenths of a milliliter, the resulting answer will be within the 10% allowable difference.

For the purpose of consistency throughout the remainder of this book, all computations will use 1 milliliter equivalent to 15 minims.

Change

$$40 \text{ ml to drams.}$$

This means

$$40 \text{ ml} = \underline{\hspace{1cm}} ʒ$$

First, determine a ratio from the given information:

$$\frac{x\ ʒ}{40 \text{ ml}}$$

From Table 2.4 determine an equivalence using milliliters and drams:

$$4 \text{ ml} = 1\ ʒ$$

Use this equivalence to set up a second ratio (be sure the same units appear in the numerator and denominator of both ratios):

$$\frac{1\ ʒ}{4 \text{ ml}}$$

ʒ should be in the numerator and ml in the denominator because the first ratio is set up with these units

Once the two ratios are determined, set them equal:

$$\frac{x\ 3}{40\ ml} = \frac{1\ 3}{4\ ml}$$

Use the numerical values to solve for x:

$$\frac{x}{40} = \frac{1}{4}$$

$$4x = 40(1)$$

$$4x = 40$$

$$\frac{\cancel{4}x}{\cancel{4}} = \frac{40}{4}$$

$$x = \frac{40}{4} = 10$$

The correct answer is 10 drams; that is,

$$40\ ml = 10\ 3$$

EXAMPLE 2.16

$$2\ ml = \underline{\hspace{1.5cm}}\ \mathfrak{m}$$

1. From the given problem complete the ratio: $\dfrac{\boxed{}\ ml}{\boxed{}\ \mathfrak{m}}$

2. Choose an equivalence for milliliters and minims from Table 2.4.

3. Write a ratio using the information in step 2.

4. Set the two ratios equal.

5. Solve for the unknown value.

EXAMPLE 2.17

$$gr\ \frac{1}{4} = \underline{\hspace{1.5cm}}\ mg$$

1. Use information in the problem and in Table 2.4 to determine a proportion (check before solving).

2. Solve for the unknown value.

Exercise 20

1. ʒ ii = _____ g

2. ʒ T = _____ ml

3. Change gr $\frac{1}{8}$ to milligrams

4. How many drops in 3 ml?

5. 25 ℥ = _____ ml

6. Change 45 ml to ounces.

Although the proportion method for changing units applies uniformly to all changes between systems, applying rules is often a more expedient method for performing conversions. Rules for common conversions are presented below. But remember that if a required unit change does not directly fit a rule, the proportion method should be used.

RULE 1: *Grams to grains* To change grams to grains, multiply the number of grams by 15.

RULE 2: *Grains to grams* To change grains to grams, divide the number of grains by 15.

EXAMPLE 2.18

$$3 \text{ g} = \text{_____ gr}$$

1. Changing _____ to _____ , use Rule _____ .
2. Number of grams = _____ .
3. Solve for the unknown.

EXAMPLE 2.19

$$\text{gr } \frac{1}{4} = \text{_____ g}$$

1. Changing _____ to _____ , use Rule _____ .
2. Number of grains = _____ .
3. Find the number of grams.

Exercise 21

1. 0.2 g = _____ gr

2. gr $\frac{1}{15}$ = _____ g

3. 0.03 gr = _____ gr

4. gr xv = _____ g

RULE 3: *Grains to milligrams* To change grains to milligrams, multiply the number of grains by 60.

RULE 4: *Milligrams to grains* To change milligrams to grains, divide the number of milligrams by 60.

EXAMPLE 2.20

$$30 \text{ mg} = \underline{\hspace{1cm}} \text{gr}$$

1. Changing _____ to _____ , use Rule _____ .
2. Number of milligrams = _____ .
3. Find the number of grains.

EXAMPLE 2.21

$$\text{gr} \frac{1}{2} = \underline{\hspace{1cm}} \text{mg}$$

1. Changing _____ to _____ , use Rule _____ .
2. Number of grains = _____ .
3. Find the number of milligrams.

Exercise 22

1. $\text{gr} \frac{1}{4} = \underline{\hspace{1cm}} \text{mg}$

2. $0.25 \text{ mg} = \underline{\hspace{1cm}} \text{gr}$

3. $\text{gr} \frac{1}{300} = \underline{\hspace{1cm}} \text{mg}$

4. $3 \text{ mg} = \underline{\hspace{1cm}} \text{gr}$

RULE 5: *Ounces to grams*   To change ounces to grams, multiply the number of ounces by 30.

RULE 6: *Grams to ounces*   To change grams to ounces, divide the number of grams by 30.

EXAMPLE 2.22

$$60 \text{ g} = \underline{\hspace{1cm}} ℥$$

1. Changing _____ to _____ , use Rule _____ .
2. How many grams?
3. Find the number of ounces.

EXAMPLE 2.23

$$℥ \text{ iss} = \underline{\hspace{1cm}} \text{g}$$

1. Changing _____ to _____ , use Rule _____ .
2. How many ounces?
3. Find the number of grams.

Exercise 23

    1. 30 g = _____ ℥   **2.** 150 g = _____ ℥

    3. ℥ iii = _____ g   **4.** ℥ ss = _____ g

    RULE 7: *Milliliters* to minims*   To change milliliters to minims, multiply the number of milliliters by 15.

    RULE 8: *Minims to milliliters**   To change minims to milliliters, divide the number of minims by 15.

EXAMPLE 2.24

$$3 \text{ ml} = \underline{\hspace{2cm}} \; ♍$$

    1. Changing _____ to _____ , use Rule _____ .
    2. Number of milliliters = _____ .
    3. Find the number of minims.

EXAMPLE 2.25

$$♍ \text{ xviii} = \underline{\hspace{2cm}} \; \text{ml}$$

    1. Changing _____ to _____ , use Rule _____ .
    2. Number of minims = _____ .
    3. Find the number of milliliters.

Exercise 24

    1. $\frac{3}{4}$ ml = _____ ♍   **2.** ♍ xvi = _____ ml

    3. 0.9 ml = _____ ♍   **4.** ♍ xxx = _____ ml

    RULE 9: *Ounces to milliliters**   To change ounces to milliliters, multiply the number of ounces by 30.

    RULE 10: *Milliliters* to ounces*   To change milliliters to ounces, divide the number of milliliters by 30.

EXAMPLE 2.26

$$75 \text{ ml} = \underline{\hspace{2cm}} \; ℥$$

    1. Changing _____ to _____ , use Rule _____ .
    2. Number of milliliters = _____ .
    3. Find the number of ounces.

---

*Recall that 1 ml = 1 cc, that is, the word milliliter may be replaced by cubic centimeter (cc).

EXAMPLE 2.27

$$\text{℥ ss} = \underline{\hspace{2cm}} \text{ml}$$

1. Changing _____ to _____ , use Rule _____ .
2. Number of ounces = _____ .
3. Find the number of milliliters.

Exercise 25

1. ℥ c = _____ ml   2. 25 ml = _____ ℥

3. ℥ i = _____ ml   4. 150 ml = _____ ℥

Occasionally weight measured in pounds needs to be changed to the equivalent value in kilograms and vice versa. This pound weight is in the Avoirdupois system. In this system, 2.2 pounds is equivalent to 1 kilogram.

RULE 11: *Kilograms to pounds* To change kilograms to pounds, multiply the number of kilograms by 2.2

RULE 12: *Pounds to kilograms* To change pounds to kilograms, divide the number of pounds by 2.2.

EXAMPLE 2.28

$$11 \text{ kg} = \underline{\hspace{2cm}} \text{lb}$$

1. Changing _____ to _____ , use Rule _____ .
2. Number of kilograms = _____ .
3. Find the number of pounds.

EXAMPLE 2.29

$$19.8 \text{ lb} = \underline{\hspace{2cm}} \text{kg}$$

1. Changing _____ to _____ , use Rule _____ .
2. Number of pounds = _____ .
3. Find the number of kilograms.

Exercise 26

Solve the following. Express answers to the nearest tenth of a unit.

1. 3 kg = _____ lb

2. 20 lb = _____ kg

3. 14 kg = _____ lb

4. 53.4 lb = _____ kg

5. 24.3 kg = _____ lb

6. 37.5 lb = _____ kg

TEMPERATURE EQUIVALENTS

Temperature is measured using two scales: Fahrenheit and Celsius. The relationship between the scales is:

	Fahrenheit	Celsius
boiling	212	100
freezing	32	0

The Celsius scale was an effort to obtain a scale where freezing was 0 and boiling was 100.

RULE 13: *Fahrenheit to Celsius*   To change Fahrenheit to Celsius, subtract 32 from the number. Then divide the resulting difference by 1.8.

$$C = \frac{(F - 32)}{1.8}$$

RULE 14: *Celsius to Fahrenheit*   To change Celsius to Fahrenheit, multiply the number by 1.8. Then add 32 to the resulting product.

$$F = 1.8 (C) + 32$$

EXAMPLE 2.30

Solve the following.

$$78\ F = \underline{\hspace{1cm}} C$$

1. Changing _____ to _____ , use Rule _____ .
2. Number of degrees Fahrenheit = _____ .
3. Find the number of degrees Celsius.

EXAMPLE 2.31

Solve the following.

$$17\ C = \underline{\hspace{1cm}} F$$

1. Changing _____ to _____ , use Rule _____ .
2. Number of degrees Celsius = _____ .
3. Find the number of degrees Fahrenheit.

Exercise 27

Solve the following. Express answers to the nearest tenth of a degree.

1. 15 C = _____ F

2. 82.4 F = _____ C

3. 3 C = _____ F

4. 68 F = _____ C

5. 37 C = _____ F

6. 14 F = _____ C

Exercise 28

These problems review the conversions learned in this chapter. Solve using proportions:

1. gtt xv = _____ ♏

2. 7 g = _____ gr

3. ℥ vii = _____ T

4. 50 mg = _____ gr

Solve by applying the correct rule:

5. ℥ 1   = _____ ml

6. ℥ xvi = _____ g

7. ♏ 24 = _____ ml

8. gr xxx = _____ g

9. gr $\frac{1}{6}$ = _____ mg

10. ♏ xx = _____ ml

11. 50 ml = _____ ℥

12. ♏ xxx = _____ gtt

13. 4 mg = _____ gr

14. gr $\frac{3}{8}$ = _____ mg

15. 100 g = _____ ℥

16. 5 g   = _____ gr

17. ℥ i   = _____ g

18. 90 g = _____ ℥

19. 75 ml = _____ ℥

20. 4 g   = _____ gr

21. 0.4 ml = _____ ♏

22. ℥ ii = _____ ml

23. 45 mg _____ gr

24. 0.5 ml = _____ ♏

25. 50 F = _____ C

26. 7 C   = _____ F

27. −2 C = _____ F

28. 102 F = _____ C

29. 98.6 F = _____ C

30. −11 C = _____ F

ANSWERS TO EXAMPLES

Example 2.1

18 ml
4 centiliters
5 cg
7 m
2 kg
3 deciliters
5 centimeters

Example 2.2

1. $\dfrac{x \text{ liters}}{450 \text{ ml}}$

2. 1 liter $=$ 1000 ml

3. $\dfrac{1 \text{ liter}}{1000 \text{ ml}}$

4. $\dfrac{x \text{ liters}}{450 \text{ ml}} = \dfrac{1 \text{ liter}}{1000 \text{ ml}}$

5. $\dfrac{x}{450} = \dfrac{1}{1000}$

   $1000x = 450$

   $x = \dfrac{450}{1000} = 0.45$ liter

Example 2.3

$\dfrac{x \text{ mg}}{38 \text{ g}}$

We know 1 g $=$ 1000 mg

$\dfrac{1000 \text{ mg}}{1 \text{ g}}$

$\dfrac{x \text{ mg}}{38 \text{ g}} = \dfrac{1000 \text{ mg}}{1 \text{ g}}$

$\dfrac{x}{38} = \dfrac{1000}{1}$

$x = 38{,}000$ mg

Example 2.4

$\dfrac{54 \text{ cm}}{x \text{ m}}$

We know 1 m $=$ 100 cm

$\dfrac{54}{x \text{ m}} = \dfrac{100 \text{ cm}}{1 \text{ m}}$

$\dfrac{54}{x} = \dfrac{100}{1}$

$100x = 54$

$x = \dfrac{54}{100}$

$x = 0.54$ m

Example 2.5

6000 ml
300 ml
7000 mg
15000 mm

Example 2.6

0.750 liter
9.8 g
0.042 m

Example 2.7

4000 g
4230 g
543 g
2570 m

Example 2.8

1.545 kg
0.045 kl
0.137 km

Example 2.9

2. 9 drams
3. 5 ounces
4. $1\frac{1}{2}$ grains
5. $\frac{1}{4}$ grain

Example 2.10

1. $7\frac{1}{2}$ fluidrams
2. $\frac{1}{2}$ pint
3. 4 fluidounces
4. 3 gallons
5. 5 minims

Example 2.11

1. $\frac{x\,f\!\!\mathfrak{z}}{2\,f\!\!\mathfrak{z}}$
2. $1\,f\!\!\mathfrak{z} = 8\,f\!\!\mathfrak{z}$
3. $\frac{1\,f\!\!\mathfrak{z}}{8\,f\!\!\mathfrak{z}}$
4. $\frac{x\,f\!\!\mathfrak{z}}{2\,f\!\!\mathfrak{z}} = \frac{1\,f\!\!\mathfrak{z}}{8\,f\!\!\mathfrak{z}}$
5. $\frac{x}{2} = \frac{1}{8}$

$8x = 2$

$x = \frac{2}{8} = \frac{1}{4}$

$\frac{1}{4}\,f\!\!\mathfrak{z}$

Example 2.12

1. $\frac{x\,f\!\!\mathfrak{z}}{3\,qt}$
2. $1\,qt = 2\,pt = 2(16\,f\!\!\mathfrak{z}) = 32\,f\!\!\mathfrak{z}$
3. $\frac{32\,f\!\!\mathfrak{z}}{1\,qt}$
4. $\frac{x\,f\!\!\mathfrak{z}}{3\,qt} = \frac{32\,f\!\!\mathfrak{z}}{1\,qt}$
5. $\frac{x}{3} = \frac{32}{1}$

$x = 3(32) = 96$

$96\,f\!\!\mathfrak{z}$

Example 2.13

1. Rule 1
2. 8
3. $1\frac{1}{2}$
4. $1\frac{1}{2} \times 8 = 12$ drams

Example 2.14

1. Rule 2
2. 60
3. 120
4. $120 \div 60 = 2\,\mathfrak{z}$

Example 2.15

1. $\frac{3\,oz}{x\,gtt}$
2. $\frac{1\,oz}{360\,gtt}$
3. $\frac{3\,oz}{x\,gtt} = \frac{1\,oz}{360\,gtt}$
4. $\frac{3}{x} = \frac{1}{360}$

$x = 3(360) = 1080\,gtt$

Example 2.16

1. $\frac{2\,ml}{x\,\mathfrak{m}}$
2. $1\,ml = 15\,\mathfrak{m}$
3. $\frac{1\,ml}{15\,\mathfrak{m}}$
4. $\frac{2\,ml}{x\,\mathfrak{m}} = \frac{1\,ml}{15\,\mathfrak{m}}$
5. $\frac{2}{x} = \frac{1}{15}$

$x = 2(15) = 30$

$30\,\mathfrak{m}$

Example 2.17

$\frac{x\,mg}{\frac{1}{4}\,gr} = \frac{60\,mg}{1\,gr}$

$\frac{x}{\frac{1}{4}} = \frac{60}{1}$

$x = \frac{1}{4}(60)$

$x = 15\,mg$

Example 2.18

1. grams to grains, Rule 1
2. 3
3. $3(15) = 45\,gr$

Example 2.19
1. grains to grams, Rule 2
2. $\frac{1}{4}$
3. $\frac{1}{4} \div 15 = \frac{1}{4} \times \frac{1}{15} = \frac{1}{60}$

   $\frac{1}{60}$ g

Example 2.20
1. milligrams to grains, Rule 4
2. 30
3. $30 \div 60 = \frac{1}{2}$

   $\frac{1}{2}$ gr

Example 2.21
1. grains to milligrams, Rule 3
2. $\frac{1}{2}$
3. $\frac{1}{2}(60) = 30$

   30 mg

Example 2.22
1. grams to ounces, Rule 6
2. 60
3. $60 \div 30 = 2$
   2 ounces

Example 2.23
1. ounces to grams, Rule 5
2. $1\frac{1}{2}$
3. $\left(1\frac{1}{2}\right)(30) = (1.5)(30) = 45$

   45 g

Example 2.24
1. milliliters to minims, Rule 7
2. 73
3. $3(15) = 45$
   45 ℳ

Example 2.25
1. minims to milliliters, Rule 8
2. 18
3. $18 \div 15 = \frac{18}{15} = \frac{6}{5}$

   $\frac{6}{5}$ ml = 1.2 ml

Example 2.26
1. milliliters to ounces, Rule 10
2. 75
3. $75 \div 30 = 2.5$
   2.5 ℥

Example 2.27
1. ounces to milliliters, Rule 9
2. $\frac{1}{2}$
3. $\frac{1}{2} \times 30 = 15$
   15 ml

Example 2.28
1. kilograms to pounds, Rule 11
2. 11
3. $11(2.2) = 24.2$ lbs

Example 2.29
1. pounds to kilograms, Rule 12
2. 19.8
3. $19.8 \div 2.2 = 9$ kg

Example 2.30
1. Fahrenheit to Celsius, Rule 13
2. 78
3. $\frac{(78 - 32)}{1.8} = \frac{46}{1.8} = 25.6$ C

Example 2.31
1. Celsius to Fahrenheit, Rule 14
2. 17
3. $1.8(17) + 3 = 62.6$ F

Unit 2 consists of chapters dealing with medication computations associated with the different situations encountered by the nurse, such as pediatric medications, oral medications, intramuscular medications, or intravenous medications. The majority of the problems appearing in this unit were taken from actual physician orders while the remainder of the problems were chosen to provide additional practice with the applied mathematical techniques.

The mathematical problem originates with the drug order and the label on the vial. It is from these two sources that the nurse obtains the information used in the mathematical computations. Nurses usually refer to the drug order as the "desired" dosage and to the drug label information as the "on-hand" dosage.

To simulate the nurse's functioning as it relates to mathematical computations, the drug order and drug label have been used in the chapters in this unit. No two companies use exactly the same form for their labels, so a generic form is used in this book. The drug order, on the other hand, has been more of a problem to simulate. Some nursing practice environments still use a drug card and kardex, other situations use a unit-dose format, and computerized drug orders are used in some nursing practice situations. All of these are merely different formats used toward the same goal: communicating the physician's order for medication for a specific patient. Most nursing environments are currently implementing some form of computerized format for managing medication information. Therefore the authors have chosen to present drug orders using a drug order printout format.

Drug Order Printout

Name: Lewis, George	**Room:** 204
Medication:	
Kantrex 500 mg	
Route: I.M.	**Time:** bid

There also seem to be some arbitrary "rules of thumb" regarding the appropriate equivalents for 1 milliliter. Sometimes the equivalent used is 1 ml = 15 minims, while at other times 1 ml = 16 minims. To accurately calculate and provide answers in this text, 1 ml = 15 minims is used in all exercises. It should be noted that within the 10% tolerance for allowable error, the computed answer should make negligible difference in the answers. When working problems, remember to use

$$1 \text{ ml} = 15 \text{ minims}$$

3 ORAL MEDICATIONS

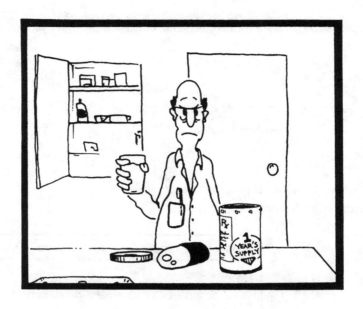

CHAPTER OBJECTIVES

- Use the basic operations of ratio and proportions to solve problems for the oral medications
- Demonstrate proficiency in correctly reading medication labels
- Exhibit proficiency in correctly reading medication orders
- Demonstrate proficiency in correctly interpreting medicine cup measurement scales
- Display proficiency in simulating desired volume of liquid medication on standard medicine cups

INTRODUCTION

Oral administration is one of the most common methods of administering medicine in hospitals today. Therefore in many schools of nursing the student begins the administration of medicines with the oral route. Other methods for administering medications will be discussed in later chapters.

Often the medication you have on hand will be of a different dosage from the one ordered by the physician. When this occurs, the nurse performs some mathematical computations to determine what amount of the drug on hand is needed to give the patient the dosage ordered by the physician.

The following examples should help you develop a method for solving dosage problems encountered with oral medications.

TABLETS

The physician has ordered propranolol hydrochloride 10 mg. The label indicates each tablet contains 20 mg.

The drug on hand is 20 mg per tablet; desired dosage is 10 mg. Set up a proportion and use the ideas discussed in Chapter 1 to compute the correct dosage.

On hand   Desired

$$\frac{1 \text{ tablet}}{20 \text{ mg}} \qquad \frac{x \text{ tablets}}{10 \text{ mg}}$$

The two ratios, on hand and desired, are set up so that the numerator and denominator units correspond: tablets to milligrams in each case

Now that two ratios are formed, set them equal and solve for the value of x.

Step			If trouble going from step to step		Go to page
1	$\frac{1}{20} = \frac{x}{10}$				
2	$20x = 10$	now divide each side by 20	1	2	35
3	$x = \frac{10}{20}$	perform the division	2	3	37
4	$x = \frac{1}{2}$ tab		3	4	12

So $\frac{1}{2}$ tablet constitutes the correct dosage.

Read the following order:

Name: J. Doe	**Room:** 18
Medication:
Codeine 30 mg every 4 hrs prn
Route: oral

Secure the codeine tablets for J. Doe. The label reads codeine sulfate 60 mg.

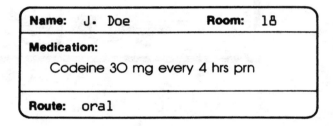

Since the dosage on the drug order (*desired* dosage) and the dosage on the drug label (*on-hand* dosage) are not the same, a computation is necessary.

The drug on hand is 60 mg per tablet. The desired dosage is 30 mg. Setting up a proportion, again use the ideas in Chapter 1.

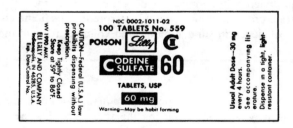

On hand   Desired

$$\frac{1 \text{ tablet}}{60 \text{ mg}} \qquad \frac{x \text{ tablets}}{30 \text{ mg}}$$

Step		If trouble going from step to step		Go to page
1	$\frac{1}{60} = \frac{x}{30}$			
2	$60x = 30(1)$	1	2	35
3	$x = \frac{30}{60}$	2	3	37
4	$x = \frac{1}{2}$ tab	3	4	12

If you had trouble obtaining $\frac{1}{2}$ tablet as the correct dosage, review the appropriate math review section.

For your benefit, the arithmetic computation involved in each step of the solution is outlined with reference to Chapter 1.

Work the following example.

EXAMPLE 3.1*

Drug Order Printout

Name: J. Doe	**Room:** 8
Medication: aspirin gr xv	
Route: oral	**Time:** q 6 h prn

Drug Label

N 0047-0606-32

6505-00-153-8750

Aspirin Tablets, USP

Analgesic/Antipyretic

For relief of minor aches and pains and reduction of fever.

WARNING: Children and teenagers should not use this medicine for chicken pox or flu symptoms before a doctor is consulted about Reye syndrome, a rare but serious illness.

Ingredients: Aspirin. Also contains corn starch; microcrystalline cellulose.

Quality Sealed for your protection*

1000 Tablets
5 grains (325 mg) each

W|C   WARNER CHILCOTT

---

* Answers to examples appear on pages 96-98.

1. What is the drug dosage on hand? _____
2. What is the drug dosage desired? _____
3. Set up the proportion by filling the boxes with the missing information.

On hand   Desired

$\dfrac{\boxed{} \text{ tablets}}{5 \text{ gr}}$ $\dfrac{x \text{ tablets}}{\boxed{} \text{ gr}}$

4. Set up the proportion and solve for x.

5. How many tablets is the nurse to give? _____

EXAMPLE 3.2

As the medicine nurse, you find the following drug order and drug label:

Drug Order Printout

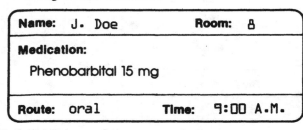

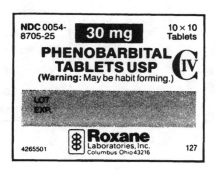

In the space below, determine the correct dosage to be administered. Work Example 3.2 here (when finished, check work in the answers section).

EXAMPLE 3.3

The physician orders Lanoxin 0.5 mg. The drug label reads Lanoxin 0.25 mg. How many tablets should the patient receive?

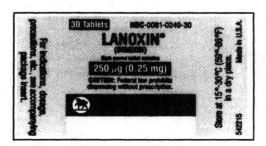

The physician orders Gantrisin gr xv. The label reads Gantrisin 250 mg.

Reading the drug order and drug label, your attention first focuses on the dose. The drug order is expressed in the apothecaries' system (gr xv), and the drug label is in the metric system (250 mg). First, determine an equivalency of units so that a proportion can be set up using like units for on hand and desired dosages.

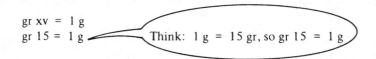

gr xv = 1 g
gr 15 = 1 g

Think: 1 g = 15 gr, so gr 15 = 1 g

Set up the ratios:

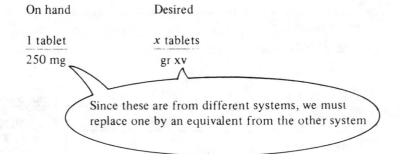

On hand	Desired
$\dfrac{1 \text{ tablet}}{250 \text{ mg}}$	$\dfrac{x \text{ tablets}}{\text{gr xv}}$

Since these are from different systems, we must replace one by an equivalent from the other system

Replace gr xv by 1 g because 15 gr = 1 g.

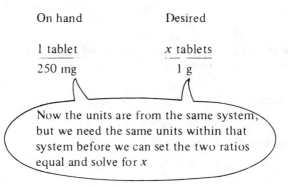

On hand	Desired
$\dfrac{1 \text{ tablet}}{250 \text{ mg}}$	$\dfrac{x \text{ tablets}}{1 \text{ g}}$

Now the units are from the same system, but we need the same units within that system before we can set the two ratios equal and solve for x

Recall that 1 g is 1000 mg (to change grams to milligrams, move the decimal three places to the right, so 1 g = 1000 mg). When 1 g is replaced by its equivalent, the proportion becomes

On hand	Desired
$\dfrac{1 \text{ tablet}}{250 \text{ mg}}$	$\dfrac{x \text{ tablets}}{1000 \text{ mg}}$

Since the units in the two ratios are identical, set the ratios equal and solve:

$$\frac{1}{250} = \frac{x}{1000}$$

$$250x = 1000$$

$$x = \frac{1000}{250} = 4$$

Four tablets, each containing 250 mg, will provide your patient with gr xv.

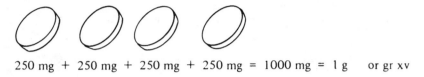

250 mg + 250 mg + 250 mg + 250 mg = 1000 mg = 1 g   or gr xv

EXAMPLE 3.4

Read the following drug order and drug label:

Name: J. Doe	Room: 13
Medication:	
phenobarbital gr ss	
Route: oral	**Time:** 9/1/6

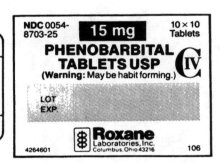

NDC 0054-8703-25   **15 mg**   10 × 10 Tablets

PHENOBARBITAL TABLETS USP C IV
(Warning: May be habit forming.)

LOT
EXP.

Roxane Laboratories, Inc.
Columbus, Ohio 43216

4264601   106

1. Use the information on the drug order and drug label to set up a proportion (but check your equation before solving).

2. Solve the equation to determine the dosage.

LIQUIDS

The past few examples have dealt specifically with oral medications involving tablets. This section will focus on dosage for liquid medications. The physician orders Mellaril concentrate 60 mg. The nurse finds Mellaril concentrate 30 mg/ml in the drug cabinet. How much Mellaril should the nurse administer?

To compute the dosage, first check the drug available:

On hand

30 mg in 1 ml

The dosage requested by the physician should be considered next:

Desired

60 mg in ? ml

It is realized that 60 mg is requested, but the number of milliliters required to contain the 60 mg is not known. This has been represented above by a question mark. Liquid medication problems are similar to the tablet medications; indeed, the methods of solving the two types of problems are identical.

Set up the proportion as in the previous examples:

On hand	Desired
$\dfrac{1 \text{ ml}}{30 \text{ mg}}$	$\dfrac{x \text{ ml}}{60 \text{ mg}}$

$$\frac{1}{30} = \frac{x}{60}$$
$$30x = 60 \ (1)$$
$$x = \frac{60}{30} = 2 \text{ ml}$$

The necessary dosage is 2 ml.

Is this answer reasonable? Yes, when you think that

$$\text{add} \quad \frac{\begin{array}{l}1 \text{ ml contains } 30 \text{ mg} \quad \text{and}\\ 1 \text{ ml contains } 30 \text{ mg}\end{array}}{}$$

yields   2 ml contains 60 mg

So the procedure works for both tablets and liquid medications.

Work the following example.

EXAMPLE 3.5

The physician orders elixir of phenobarbital 4 mg. The bottle in the drug cabinet reads 4 mg/5 ml. How much elixir of phenobarbital must the nurse give to ensure correct dosage?

1. On hand   Desired

$$\frac{5 \text{ ml}}{4 \text{ mg}}$$

Is milliliters the usual unit of measure? _____

2. Set up the proportion to solve the problem.

On hand   Desired

$$\frac{5 \text{ ml}}{4 \text{ mg}} \qquad \frac{\boxed{} \text{ ml}}{\boxed{}}$$

$$\frac{5}{4} = \frac{\boxed{}}{\boxed{}}$$

3. Check the above equation before you solve.
4. Solve the equation.

5. What is the correct dosage? _____

In the above example, did you realize that a mathematical computation was not necessary because both the on-hand and desired dosages were identical? When the desired and on-hand drugs are the same measure (4 mg), the number of units of volume (5 ml) on the drug label constitutes the correct dosage.

Read the following drug order and drug label:

Drug Order Printout

Name: J. Doe   **Room:** 12

Medication:
    Benadryl elixir 25 mg

Route: oral   **Time:** 6/12/6/12

Drug Label

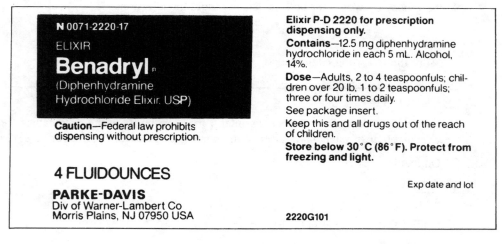

Set up the proportion to determine the correct dosage:

	On hand	Desired
	$\dfrac{12.5 \text{ mg}}{5 \text{ ml}}$	$\dfrac{25 \text{ mg}}{x \text{ ml}}$

Step		If trouble going from step to step	Go to page
1	$\dfrac{12.5}{5} = \dfrac{25}{x}$		
2	$12.5x = 125$	1 2	35
3	$x = \dfrac{125}{12.5}$	2 3	37
4	$x = 10$	3 4	12

The correct dosage is 10 ml.

EXAMPLE 3.6

Drug Order Printout

Drug Label

Name: J. Doe	**Room:** 2
Medication: Erythromycin 400 mg	
Route: oral	**Time:** 6/12/6

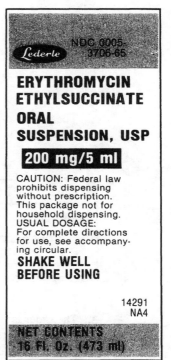

ERYTHROMYCIN ETHYLSUCCINATE ORAL SUSPENSION, USP

200 mg/5 ml

CAUTION: Federal law prohibits dispensing without prescription. This package not for household dispensing. USUAL DOSAGE: For complete directions for use, see accompanying circular.

SHAKE WELL BEFORE USING

14291 NA4

NET CONTENTS 16 Fl. Oz. (473 ml)

1. What is the dose of
   a. The drug on hand? _____
   b. The drug desired? _____
2. Now set up a proportion to determine the correct dosage:

On hand	Desired
$\dfrac{5 \text{ ml}}{\boxed{} \text{ mg}}$	$\dfrac{\boxed{} \text{ ml}}{400 \text{ mg}}$

$$\frac{5}{\boxed{}} = \frac{\boxed{}}{400}$$

3. Solve for the unknown number of milliliters.

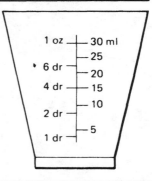

4. Mark the correct dosage on the medicine cup.

If you had difficulty in the above example, review the problem worked immediately preceding the example. If you still have difficulty, review the entire chapter before attempting the exercises.

Exercise 29

DIRECTIONS: Some of the following problems will require you to extract information from drug orders and drug labels. For all problems compute the correct dosage. When a medicine cup is given, shade the medicine cup to indicate your answer.

1. The order is for Tylenol elixir 120 mg. The drug label reads Tylenol elixir 120 mg/5 ml. How many milliliters does the patient receive? _____

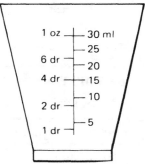

2. The physician orders ferrous sulfate 500 mg. The drug label reads ferrous sulfate 220 mg/5 ml. How many milliliters of ferrous sulfate does the patient receive? _____

Drug Order Printout

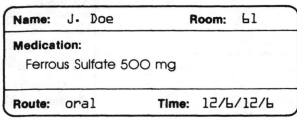

Name: J. Doe	**Room:** 61
Medication: Ferrous Sulfate 500 mg	
Route: oral	**Time:** 12/6/12/6

3. The order is for Pen-Vee K 250 mg. The drug label reads Pen-Vee K 125 mg/5 ml. How many milliliters does the patient receive? _____

ART

4.

Name:	J. Doe	**Room:**	30

Medication:

Synthroid 0.1 mg

Route:	oral	**Time:**	stat

Drug Label

BOOTS-FLINT

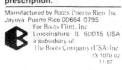

SYNTHROID®
(Levothyroxine Sodium
Tablets, USP)

100 mcg (0.1 mg)

Dosage. Adults: Initial - 25 to 100 mcg
(0.025 to 0.1 mg) daily. Usual mainte-
nance dose - 100 to 200 mcg (0.1 to 0.2
mg) daily. Children: Initial - 25 mcg
(0.025 mg) daily. Dosage adjusted by
physician until desired response is obtained. See directions for higher main-
tenance dosage. SEE ACCOMPANYING
DIRECTIONS
Contains FD&C Yellow No. 5 (tartrazine)
as a color additive
Keep this and all medications out of the
reach of children
For hospital use only. Packaging is not
child resistant
**Caution: Federal (U.S.A.) law
prohibits dispensing without
prescription.**

Manufactured by Boots Puerto Rico, Inc.
Jayuya, Puerto Rico 00664 0795
For Boots Flint, Inc.
Lincolnshire, IL 60015 USA
a subsidiary of
The Boots Company (USA) Inc.
13 1070 02
11-87

How many tablets of synthroid does the patient receive? _____

5. The order is for Nembutal elixir 60 mg. The drug label reads Nembutal elixir 20 mg/5 ml.
How many milliliters of Nembutal elixir does the patient receive? _____

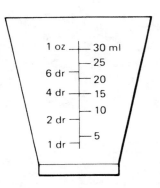

6. The order is for Feosol elixir 300 mg. The drug label reads Feosol elixir 220 mg/5 ml. How many milliliters does the patient receive? _____

7.   Drug Order Printout

Name: J. Doe	**Room:** 91	
Medication:		
Aldomet 250 mg		
Route: oral	**Time:** 9/5	

Drug Label

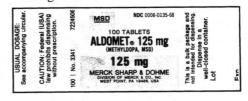

How many tablets of Aldomet does the patient receive? _____

8. The order is for chloral hydrate elixir 1 g. The drug label reads chloral hydrate elixir gr viiss/ 5 ml. How many milliliters does the patient receive? _____

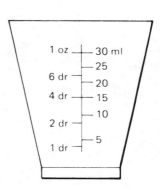

9. Drug Order Printout

Name: J. Smith   Room: 409

Medication:

Thorazine 100 mg

Route: oral   Time: 9-1-5

How many tablets should the patient receive?

Drug Label

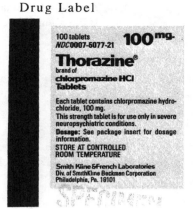

10. The physician orders Keflex suspension 250 mg. The drug label reads Keflex 125 mg/5 ml. How many milliliters should the patient receive?

11. The order is for 0.25 mg of Lanoxin elixir. The drug label reads Lanoxin elixir 0.05 mg/ml. How many milliliters should the patient receive?

12. Drug Order Printout

Name: M. Jones   Room: 101

Medication:

Thorazine 50 mg

Route: oral   Time: tid

How many tablets should the patient receive?

Drug Label

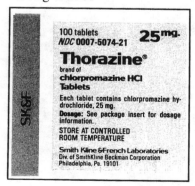

13. The physician orders Thorazine concentrate 60 mg. The drug label reads Thorazine concentrate 100 mg/ml. How many milliliters should the patient receive?

14. The physician orders leuothyroxine 100 mcg. The drug label reads leuothyroxine 200 mcg. How many tablets should the patient receive?

15. How many tablets should the patient receive?

Drug Order Printout

Name: P. Jones	**Room:** 102
Medication:	
Aspirin gr x	
Route: oral	**Time:** tid

Drug Label

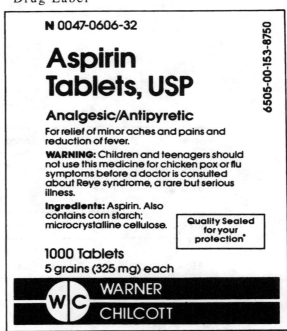

N 0047-0606-32

6505-00-153-8750

Aspirin Tablets, USP

Analgesic/Antipyretic

For relief of minor aches and pains and reduction of fever.

WARNING: Children and teenagers should not use this medicine for chicken pox or flu symptoms before a doctor is consulted about Reye syndrome, a rare but serious illness.

Ingredients: Aspirin. Also contains corn starch; microcrystalline cellulose.

Quality Sealed for your protection

1000 Tablets
5 grains (325 mg) each

WC WARNER CHILCOTT

16. The physician orders digitoxin 0.2 mg. How many tablets should the patient receive?

Drug Label

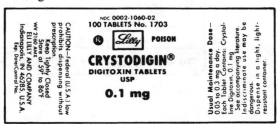

17. The order is for Ativan 2 mg. The drug label reads Ativan 1 mg. How many tablets should the patient receive?

18. The physician orders Hydrea 500 mg. How many tablets should the patient receive?

Drug Label

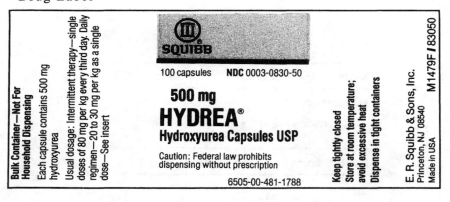

19. Drug Order Printout

Drug Label

Name:	M. Mere	Room:	601
Medication:			
Synthroid 75 mcg			
Route: oral		**Time:** daily	

How many tablets should the patient receive?

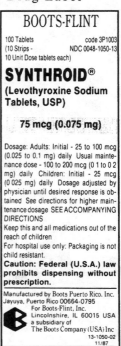

BOOTS·FLINT

100 Tablets   code 3P1003
(10 Strips -   NDC 0048-1050-13
10 Unit Dose tablets each)

SYNTHROID®

**(Levothyroxine Sodium
Tablets, USP)**

75 mcg (0.075 mg)

Dosage: Adults: Initial - 25 to 100 mcg
(0.025 to 0.1 mg) daily Usual mainte-
nance dose - 100 to 200 mcg (0 1 to 0 2
mg) daily Children: Initial - 25 mcg
(0 025 mg) daily Dosage adjusted by
physician until desired response is obtained See directions for higher main-
tenance dosage SEE ACCOMPANYING
DIRECTIONS
Keep this and all medications out of the
reach of children
For hospital use only: Packaging is not
child resistant.
**Caution: Federal (U.S.A.) law
prohibits dispensing without
prescription.**
Manufactured by Boots Puerto Rico. Inc.
Jayuya, Puerto Rico 00664-0795
For Boots-Flint, Inc.
Lincolnshire, IL 60015 USA
a subsidiary of
The Boots Company (USA) Inc
13-1050-02
11/87

20. The physician orders Gantrisin suspension 900 mg. The drug label reads Gantrisin suspension 1000 mg/10 ml. How many milliliters should the patient receive?

21. Drug Order Printout

Drug Label

Name:	P. Potter	Room:	303
Medication:			
Coumadin 10 mg			
Route: oral		**Time:** daily	

How many tablets should the patient receive?

COUMADIN ®
(crystalline warfarin sodium, U.S.P.)
5 mg
DU PONT PHARMACEUTICALS
Wilmington, Delaware 19898
Lot   YG060A
Exp.   8/89

22.   Drug Order Printout

Drug Label

Name: J. Jones   **Room:**

Medication:
 Imuran 25 mg

Route: oral   **Time:**

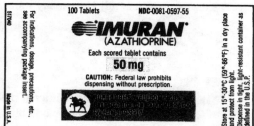

How many tablets should the patient receive?

23. The physician orders phenobarbital elixir 60 mg. The drug label reads phenobarbital elixir gr 1/4 per ml. How many milliliters should the patient receive?

24. The physician orders Ritalin 20 mg. The drug label reads Ritalin 10 mg. How many tablets should the patient receive?

25.

Name: L. Smith   **Room:**   600

Medication:
 Coumadin 2.5 mg

Route: oral   **Time:**   daily

COUMADIN ®
(crystalline warfarin sodium, U.S.P.)
5 mg
DU PONT PHARMACEUTICALS
Wilmington, Delaware 19898
Lot   YC869A
Exp.   8/89

How many tablets should the patient receive?

26. The physician orders Thorazine concentrate 60 mg. The drug label reads Thorazine concentrate 30 mg/ml. How many milliliters should the patient receive?

Exercise 30

These will give you additional practice in oral medications.

1. The order is for phenobarbital gr iss. The drug label reads phenobarbital gr ss. How many tablets should the patient receive? _____

2. The order is for Synthroid 125 mcg. The drug label reads Synthroid 0.125 mg. How many tablets should the patient receive? _____

3. The physician orders Prolixin 1 mg. The drug label reads Prolixin 2 mg. How many tablets does the patient receive? _____

4. The physician orders Aldomet 500 mg. The drug label reads Aldomet 1 g. How many tablets should the patient receive?

5. The order is for Persantine 25 mg. The drug label reads Persantine 50 mg. How many tablets does the patient receive? _____

6. The physician orders furosemide oral solution 40 mg. The drug label reads furosemide 10 mg/ml. How many milliliters should the patient receive? _____

7. The order is for Lanoxin 0.5 mg. The drug label reads Lanoxin 0.25 mg. How many tablets should the patient receive? _____

8. The order is for Elavil 25 mg. The drug label reads Elavil 10 mg. How many tablets should the patient receive? _____

9. The physician orders aspirin gr x. The drug label reads aspirin 325 mg. How many tablets should the patient receive? _____

10. The order is for chloral hydrate liquid gr viiss. The drug label reads chloral hydrate gr x per dram. How many milliliters should the patient receive? _____

11. The order is for Mycostatin mouthwash 250,000 U. The drug label reads Mycostatin mouthwash 100,000 U ml. How many milliliters should the patient receive? _____

12. The order is for Lanoxin elixir 0.125 mg. The drug label reads Lanoxin elixir 0.05 mg/ml. How many milliliters should the patient receive? _____

ANSWERS TO EXAMPLES

Example 3.1

1. gr v per tablet
2. gr xv
3.

On hand	Desired
$\dfrac{1 \text{ tablet}}{5 \text{ gr}}$	$\dfrac{x \text{ tablets}}{15 \text{ gr}}$

4. $\dfrac{1}{5} = \dfrac{x}{15}$

$5x = 15$

$x = \dfrac{15}{5}$

$x = 3$

5. Since our solution was $x = 3$, we give three tablets.

Example 3.2

On hand   Desired

Step

1. $\dfrac{1 \text{ tablet}}{30 \text{ mg}}$ $\dfrac{x \text{ tablets}}{15 \text{ mg}}$

2. $30x = 15$

3. $x = \dfrac{15}{30}$ $\begin{array}{r} 0.5 \\ 30\overline{)15.0} \\ \underline{15\ 0} \end{array}$

4. $x = 0.5$ or $\dfrac{1}{2}$ tablet

If trouble going from			Go to page
step	to	step	
1		2	35
2		3	37
3		4	12

Example 3.3

On hand   Desired

$\dfrac{1 \text{ tablet}}{0.25 \text{ mg}}$ $\dfrac{x \text{ tablets}}{0.5 \text{ mg}}$

$\dfrac{1}{0.25} = \dfrac{x}{0.5}$

$0.25x = 0.5$

$x = \dfrac{0.5}{0.25} = 2$

Two tablets.

Example 3.4

1. gr ss means $\frac{1}{2}$ grain
   Recall 1 gr = 60 mg
       gr i = 60 mg
       gr ss = 30 mg

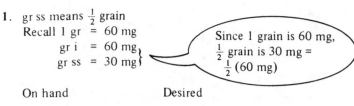

Since 1 grain is 60 mg, $\frac{1}{2}$ grain is 30 mg = $\frac{1}{2}$ (60 mg)

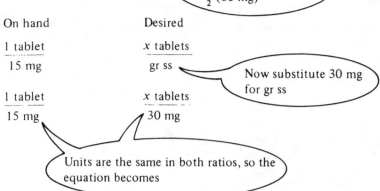

On hand   Desired

$\dfrac{1 \text{ tablet}}{15 \text{ mg}}$ $\dfrac{x \text{ tablets}}{\text{gr ss}}$

Now substitute 30 mg for gr ss

$\dfrac{1 \text{ tablet}}{15 \text{ mg}}$ $\dfrac{x \text{ tablets}}{30 \text{ mg}}$

Units are the same in both ratios, so the equation becomes

$$\frac{1}{15} = \frac{x}{30}$$

Did you get the correct equation?
If yes, return to the problem and continue as directed.
If no, review the previous exercise worked in the chapter, then rework the example again.

2. $\dfrac{1}{15} = \dfrac{x}{30}$

   $15x = 30$

   $x = \dfrac{30}{15}$

   $x = 2$

Two tablets is the correct dosage.

Example 3.5

On hand   Desired

$\dfrac{5 \text{ ml}}{4 \text{ mg}}$

1. Since the medicine cup is graduated in 5 ml increments, it is *correct* to use milliliters as the unit of measure.

2. $\dfrac{5 \text{ ml}}{4 \text{ mg}}$ $\dfrac{x \text{ ml}}{4 \text{ mg}}$

   Given as the dosage desired

3. The correct equation is

   $\dfrac{5}{4} = \dfrac{x}{4}$

4. $4x = 20$

$\quad\quad x = \frac{20}{4}$

$\quad\quad x = 5$

5. 5 ml

Example 3.6

1. a. 200 mg/5 ml   **b.** 400 mg   **4.** 10 ml

2. $\frac{5 \text{ ml}}{200 \text{ mg}}$ $\frac{x \text{ ml}}{400 \text{ mg}}$

$\quad\quad \frac{5}{200} = \frac{x}{400}$

3. $\frac{5}{200} = \frac{x}{400}$

$\quad 200x = 2000$

$\quad\quad x = \frac{2000}{200}$

$\quad\quad x = 10$

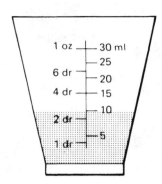

4 PARENTERAL MEDICATIONS

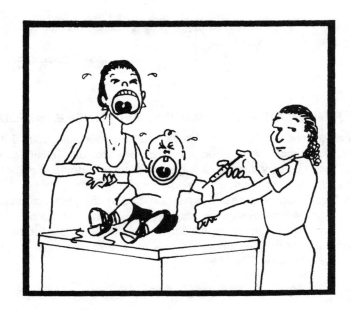

CHAPTER OBJECTIVES

- Utilize the basic operations of ratio and proportions when solving medication problems for intramuscular and subcutaneous injections
- Demonstrate proficiency in correctly reading 2½ ml syringes
- Determine dosage for medications manufactured in units
- Exhibit proficiency in accurately reading U100 syringes

INTRODUCTION

Chapter 3 dealt with oral medications. Another common method of administering medications is the parenteral route. You probably have not had many occasions to administer medications by the parenteral route before enrolling in nursing school. This method does require more specific nursing skill in that particular sites for injection must be carefully selected.

Parenteral medications are delivered by injection directly into subcutaneous tissue (subcutaneous injection), into selected muscles (intramuscular injection, abbreviated IM), or into veins (intravenous injection, abbreviated IV).

Intramuscular injection is probably the most common of the three, but nurses are assuming more and more responsibility for administering intravenous medications and solutions. Of the subcutaneous medications, insulin is probably the most common drug administered by nurses.

Because there are manufacturing differences in some drugs administered parenterally, each section begins with a short explanation of the characteristics of the drugs discussed in the section.

To correlate the arithmetical answer to the math problem with clinical applications, you will be asked to shade a syringe (such as the one pictured below) to indicate correct dosage. The amount of fluid drawn into the cylinder of the syringe is adjusted by manipulating the plunger. The plunger of the pictured syringe indicates eight-tenths of a milliliter of fluid is in the cylinder ready to be administered. For purposes of practice, the syringes used hereafter do not contain a plunger. This allows you to shade the syringe to the point where you would stop the plunger in drawing up the dosage. This simulates drawing up the medication to make the mathematical answer more meaningful.

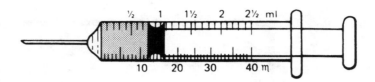

INTRAMUSCULAR MEDICATIONS FROM PREPARED-STRENGTH LIQUIDS

This section concerns intramuscular medications contained in multiple-dose vials or single-dose ampules. An ampule contains only a single dose for one injection, such as morphine 10 mg. A multiple-dose vial may contain as many as 10 doses and will specify the amount of drug contained in each milliliter of solution, e.g., morphine 10 mg/ml.

The drug dosage of prepared liquids ordered by the physician may differ from the label on the ampule or vial. When this happens, the nurse must perform a mathematical computation to determine the amount of liquid volume for the correct drug dosage. The formula for computing these dosages is the same as that used in solving dosages for oral medications.

Read the following drug order:

Name: J. Doe	Room: 2
Medication: morphine 12 mg	
Route: I.M.	**Time:** q4h prn pain

The label reads morphine 10 mg/ml. The on-hand drug is morphine, 10 milligrams per milliliter. The physician's order is for 12 mg of morphine. Set up the proportion to solve the drug problem:

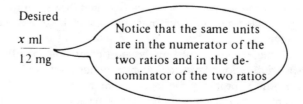

Desired

$$\frac{x \text{ ml}}{12 \text{ mg}}$$

Notice that the same units are in the numerator of the two ratios and in the denominator of the two ratios

This yields the equation

$$\frac{1}{10} = \frac{x}{12}$$

$$10x = 12 \ (1)$$

$$x = \frac{12}{10}$$

$$x = 1.2$$

The correct dosage is 1.2 ml.

To simulate drawing up the 1.2 ml of morphine, shade the syringe:

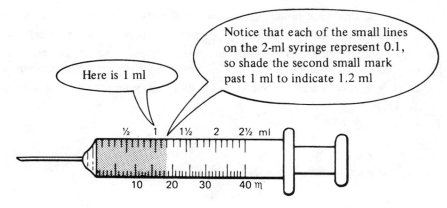

Solve the following example.

EXAMPLE 4.1*

The order is for Librium 25 mg. The label reads 100 mg in two milliliters.

1. What is the dosage on hand?
2. What is the dosage desired?
3. Set up a proportion and determine the correct dosage.

4. Shade the syringe to indicate the proper dosage.

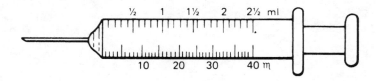

---

*Answers to examples appear on page 130.

EXAMPLE 4.2

The physician orders Nafcil 500 mg. The drug label reads Nafcil 1 g/2 ml. How many milliliters should the patient receive? _____

1. What is the dosage on hand?
2. What is the dosage desired?
3. Set up a proportion and determine the correct dosage.

Work the following problem before doing the exercises. The physician orders atropine 0.6 mg IM. The atropine vial reads atropine gr $\frac{1}{150}$ per ml. There are two avenues open at this point. Either the grains can be converted to milligrams or the milligrams can be converted to grains. As a general rule, using grains results in a more difficult math problem since the numbers involved are fractions, and so it is usually easier to convert grains to the other system of measure. Change gr $\frac{1}{150}$ to milligrams. From Table 2.4

$$\text{gr } \frac{1}{150} = 0.4 \text{ mg}$$

Set up the proportion as follows:

On hand	Desired
$\dfrac{1 \text{ ml}}{\text{gr } \frac{1}{150}}$	$\dfrac{x \text{ ml}}{0.6 \text{ mg}}$

substituting

$$\frac{1 \text{ ml}}{0.4 \text{ mg}} \qquad \frac{x \text{ ml}}{0.6 \text{ mg}}$$

The resulting equation is

$$\frac{1}{0.4} = \frac{x}{0.6}$$

$$0.4x = 0.6 \ (1)$$

$$0.4x = 0.6$$

$$x = \frac{0.6}{0.4}$$

Dividing yields

$$0.4 \overline{\smash{)}0.6\,0\ 0} \quad \begin{array}{c} 1.5 \end{array}$$

Add on zeros in case they are needed in the division

The value of x is 1.5, so the correct dosage is 1.5 ml. Syringes are marked in milliliters as a general rule, but since milliliters and cubic centimeters are equivalent,

$$1.5 \text{ ml} = 1.5 \text{ cc}$$

Hence the correct dosage is 1.5 ml or 1.5 cc. Shading the 2 ml syringe to simulate drawing up 1.5 ml yields

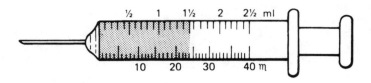

Exercise 31

DIRECTIONS: Some of the following problems will require you to extract information from drug orders and drug labels. For all problems compute the correct dosage. When a syringe is given, shade the syringe to indicate your answer.

1. The physician ordered gentamicin 60 mg IM. The drug label reads gentamicin 40 mg/ml. How many milliliters does the patient receive? _____

2. Drug Order Printout

Name: J. Doe	Room: 20
Medication:	
Kantrex 60 mg	
Route: I.M.	**Time:** 8/8

Drug Label

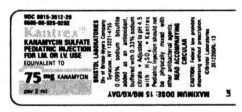

How many milliliters does the patient receive? _____

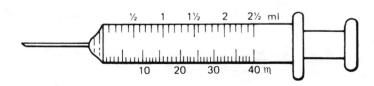

3. The physician ordered Demerol 15 mg IM. The drug label reads Demerol 50 mg/ml. How many milliliters does the patient receive? _____

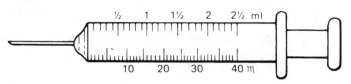

4. Drug Order Printout

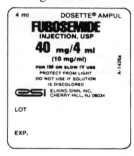

Drug Label

Name: J. Doe	**Room:** 20
Medication:	
Lasix 10 mg	
Route: I.M.	**Time:** 8/5

How many milliliters does the patient receive? _____

5. The order is for morphine 8 mg IM. The drug label reads morphine 10 mg/ml. How many milliliters does the patient receive? _____

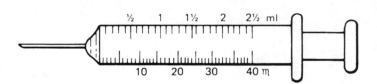

6. Drug Order Printout

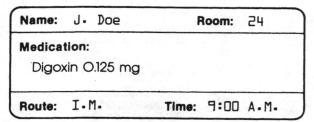

Drug Label

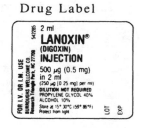

How many milliliters should the patient receive? _____

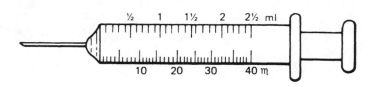

7. The order is for Dilaudid gr $\frac{1}{64}$. The drug label reads Dilaudid gr $\frac{1}{32}$ per milliliter. How many milliliters should the patient receive? _____

8. The order is for Prostaphlin 375 mg IM. How many milliliters does the patient receive? _____

Drug Label

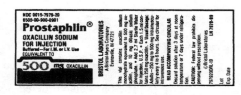

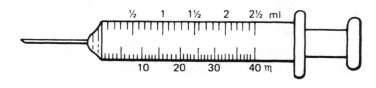

9. The order is for morphine gr $\frac{1}{6}$ IM. How many milliliters does the patient receive? _____

Drug Label

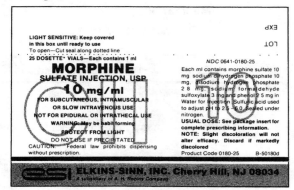

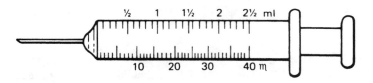

10. The order is for sodium luminal 60 mg. The label reads 130 mg/2 ml. How many milliliters does the patient receive? _____

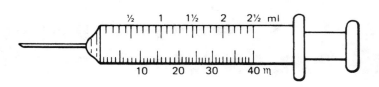

Exercise 32

These problems will give you additional practice. (Be sure to round to tenths of a milliliter.)

1. The physician ordered Serpasil 2.5 mg IM. The drug label reads Serpasil 5 mg/ml. How many milliliters should the patient receive? _____

2. The physician orders Benadryl 50 mg IM. The drug label reads Benadryl 25 mg/ml. How many milliliters does the patient receive? _____

3. The order is for Thorazine 10 mg IM. The drug label reads Thorazine 25 mg/ml. How many milliliters should the patient receive? _____

4. The physician orders Demerol 75 mg IM. The drug label reads Demerol 50 mg/ml. How many milliliters should the patient receive? _____

5. The order is for morphine 3 mg. The drug label reads morphine gr $\frac{1}{10}$ per ml. How many milliliters should the patient receive? _____

6. The physician orders digitoxin 0.3 mg. The drug label reads digitoxin 0.2 mg/ml. How many milliliters should the patient receive? _____

7. The order is for atropine gr $\frac{1}{100}$. The drug label reads atropine gr $\frac{1}{150}$ per ml. How many milliliters should the patient receive? _____

8. The order is for morphine gr $\frac{1}{12}$. The drug label reads morphine 10 mg/ml. How many milliliters should the patient receive? _____

9. The physician orders gentamicin sulfate 10 mg. The drug label reads gentamicin 40 mg/ml. How many milliliters should the patient receive? _____

10. The physician orders Demerol 75 mg. The drug label reads Demerol 100 mg in 1 milliliter. How many milliliters should the patient receive? _____

11. The physician orders Decadron 16 mg. The drug label reads Decadron 24 mg/ml. How many milliliters should the patient receive?

12. Drug Order Printout   Drug Label

Name: M. Jones	Room: 101
Medication:	
Seconal Sodium 45 mg	
Route: I.M.	**Time:** tid

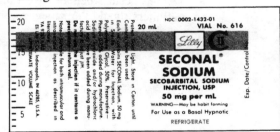

How many milliliters should the patient receive?

13. The physician orders Decadron 5 mg. The drug label reads Decadron 4 mg/ml. How many milliliters should the patient receive?

14. The physician orders Apresoline 15 mg. The drug label reads Apresoline 20 mg/ml. How many milliliters should the patient receive?

15. The physician orders Nebcin 50 mg. The drug label reads Nebcin 40 mg/ml. How many milliliters should the patient receive?

16. The physician orders Ancef 500 mg. The drug label reads Ancef 330 mg/ml. How many milliliters should the patient receive?

17. The physician orders Demerol 10 mg. The drug label reads Demerol 50 mg/ml. How many milliliters should the patient receive?

18. Drug Order Printout

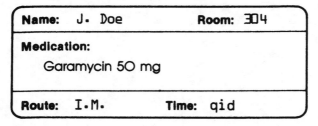

| Name: | J. Doe | Room: | 304 |

Medication:

    Garamycin 50 mg

| Route: | I.M. | Time: | qid |

Drug Label

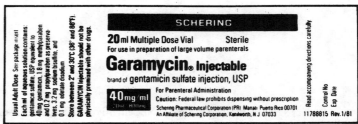

How many milliliters should the patient receive?

19. The physician orders Stadol 1 mg. The drug label reads Stadol 2 mg/ml. How many milliliters should the patient receive?

20. The physician orders Haldol 2 mg. The drug label reads Haldol 5 mg/ml. How many milliliters does the patient receive?

21. The physician orders morphine gr 1/6. How many milliliters should the patient receive?

Drug Label

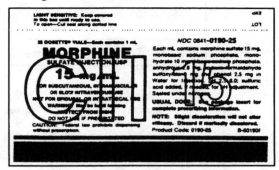

22. Drug Order Printout

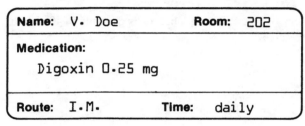

Drug Label

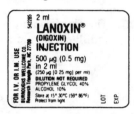

How many milliliters should the patient receive?

23. The physician orders Aqua Mephyton 5 mg. The drug label reads Aqua Mephyton 10 mg/ml. How many milliliters should the patient receive?

24. Drug Order Printout

Drug Label

Name: J. Smith	**Room:** 111
Medication: Atropine 0.1 mg	
Route: I.M.	**Time:** on call

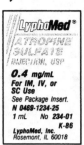

How many milliliters should the patient receive?

25. The physician orders gentamicin 10 mg. The drug label reads gentamicin 40 mg/ml. How many milliliters should the patient receive?

26. Drug Order Printout

Drug Label

Name: J. Smith	**Room:** 555
Medication: Vistaril 25 mg	
Route: I.M.	**Time:** stat

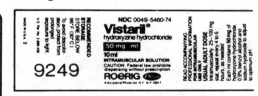

How many milliliters should the patient receive?

27. The physician orders digoxin 0.125 mg. The drug label reads digoxin 0.5 mg / 2 ml. How many milliliters should the patient receive?

28. Drug Order Printout

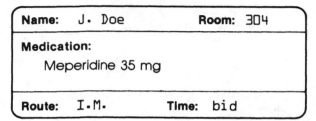

Name:	J. Doe	Room:	304

Medication:
    Meperidine 35 mg

Route:	I.M.	Time:	bid

How many milliliters should the patient receive?

Drug Label

To open – Cut seal along dotted line

NDC 0641-0150-25

25 DOSETTE· VIALS — Each contains 1 ml

MEPERIDINE

HCL INJECTION, USP

75 mg/ml

FOR INTRAMUSCULAR, SUBCUTANEOUS, OR
SLOW INTRAVENOUS USE

WARNING: May be habit forming.

Each ml contains meperidine hydrochloride 75 mg in Water for Injection with 1.5 mg sodium metabisulfite and 5 mg phenol Buffered with acetic acid—sodium acetate. Sealed under nitrogen

Caution: Federal law prohibits dispensing without prescription. **USUAL DOSE: See package insert.** Do not use if precipitated
Product Code
250150   B-50150e

ELKINS-SINN, INC. Cherry Hill, NJ 08034
A subsidiary of A. H. Robins Company

29. The physician orders atropine 0.15 mg. The drug label reads atropine 0.4 mg / ml. How many milliliters should the patient receive?

30. The physician orders Dilaudid 1 mg. The drug label reads Dilaudid gr 1/32 per ml. How many milliliters should the patient receive?

31. The physician orders Demerol 14 mg. The drug label reads Demerol 50 mg/ml. How many milliliters should the patient receive?

32. The physician orders Compazine 10 mg. The drug label reads Compazine 5 mg/ml. How many milliliters should the patient receive?

33. The physician orders atropine gr 1/300. The drug label reads atropine 0.2 mg/ml. How many milliliters should the patient receive?

34. The physician orders Vistaril 25 mg. The drug label reads Vistaril 50 mg/ml. How many milliliters should the patient receive?

35. The physician orders codeine gr 1/2. The drug label reads codeine 60 mg/ml. How many milliliters should the patient receive?

DETERMINING DOSAGE FOR DRUGS MANUFACTURED IN UNITS

Certain drugs are measured in USP units rather than in the apothecaries' or metric system. Vitamin preparations, hormones, and some antibiotics are a few examples.

One of the most common drugs measured in units is the hormone insulin. Insulin is manufactured in multiple-dose vials of U-100 strength. A U-100 vial contains 100 units of insulin per milliliter.

The insulin syringe is specifically designed for administering insulin and is calibrated in units. The insulin syringe is always a 1 ml syringe because the units (U100) are always contained in a 1 ml volume.

The physician ordering a drug manufactured in units will specify the number of units the patient should receive. It is the nurse's responsibility to determine the amount of liquid volume necessary to ensure the correct number of units for the patient.

The physician has ordered 12 U of NPH U-100 insulin to be administered each morning. Note the correct area for 12 U of U-100 insulin on the syringe below.

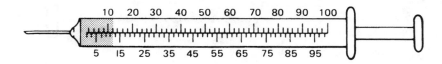

Another medication often ordered in units is heparin. The order is for 2500 U of heparin and the drug label reads heparin 5000 units per milliliter.

Drug Order Printout

Name: J. Doe	**Room:** 18
Medication:
heparin 2500 U
Route: sub q   **Time:** daily

Determine the correct dosage of heparin for administration.

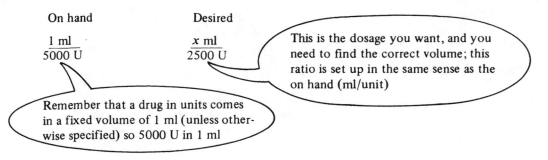

On hand

$$\frac{1 \text{ ml}}{5000 \text{ U}}$$

Desired

$$\frac{x \text{ ml}}{2500 \text{ U}}$$

This is the dosage you want, and you need to find the correct volume; this ratio is set up in the same sense as the on hand (ml/unit)

Remember that a drug in units comes in a fixed volume of 1 ml (unless otherwise specified) so 5000 U in 1 ml

This results in the equation

$$\frac{1}{5000} = \frac{x}{2500}$$

$$5000x = 2500\,(1)$$

$$x = \frac{25\cancel{00}}{50\cancel{00}} = \frac{1}{2}$$

$$x = \frac{1}{2}$$

The correct dosage is $\frac{1}{2}$ ml. Shading the correct dosage on the syringe below, we have

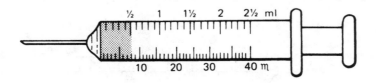

A drug commonly ordered in units is penicillin. The numbers associated with penicillin and other drugs ordered in units are usually quite large. Consider the following example using penicillin. The physician orders 150,000 U of penicillin IM. The label on the penicillin vial reads 3,000,000 U/10ml. Setting up the proportion

On hand   Desired

$$\frac{10 \text{ ml}}{3,000,000 \text{ U}} \qquad \frac{x \text{ ml}}{150,000 \text{ U}}$$

Notice the ratios are set-up in the same manner as in computation of other drugs

leads to the equation

$$\frac{10}{3,000,000} = \frac{x}{150,000}$$

$$3,000,000x = 150,000\,(10)$$

$$x = \frac{1,500,000}{3,000,000}$$

150,000 (10) = 1,500,000

$$x = \frac{1,5\cancel{00},\cancel{000}}{3,0\cancel{00},\cancel{000}}$$

canceling

$$x = \frac{15}{30} = \frac{1}{2}$$

The correct dosage is $\frac{1}{2}$ ml.

Exercise 33

DIRECTIONS: Some of the following problems will require you to extract information from drug orders and drug labels. For all problems compute the correct dosage. When a syringe is given, shade the syringe to indicate your answer.

1. The order is for heparin 12,000 U subcutaneously. The drug label reads heparin 10,000 U/ml. How many milliliters does the patient receive? _____

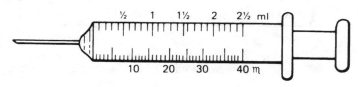

2. Drug Order Printout

Name:	J. Doe	Room:	80
Medication:			
Procaine penicillin 600,000 U			
Route: I.M.		**Time:** 9-9	

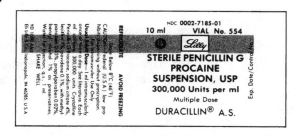

NDC 0002-7185-01
10 ml VIAL No. 554
Lilly
STERILE PENICILLIN G
PROCAINE
SUSPENSION, USP
300,000 Units per ml
Multiple Dose
DURACILLIN® A.S.

How many milliliters does the patient receive? _____

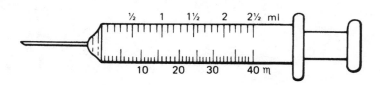

3. Drug Order Printout

Name:	J. Doe	Room:	16

Medication:

Lente insulin 35 U

Route: sub-cutaneously **Time:** 7:30

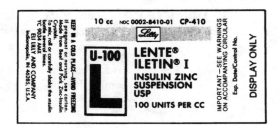

How many units of U-100 insulin does the patient receive? _____

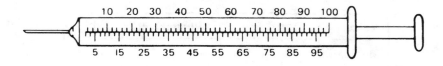

4. The physician has ordered penicillin G 600,000 U IM. The drug label reads 400,000 U/ml. How many milliliters does the patient receive? _____

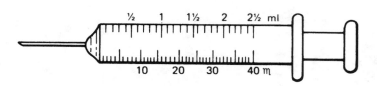

5.   Drug Order Printout   Drug Label

Name: J. Doe **Room:** 80	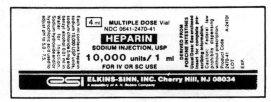
Medication: heparin 12,000 U	
Route: subcutaneous **Time:** 8/4	

How many milliliters does the patient receive? _____

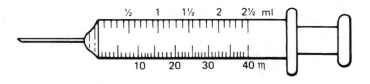

6.   The physician orders heparin 15,000 U. The drug label reads heparin 20,000 U/ml. How many milliliters should the patient receive? _____

7.   The order is for procaine penicillin 400,000 U. The drug label reads procaine penicillin 300,000 U/ml. How many milliliters does the patient receive? _____

8. Drug Order Printout   Drug Label

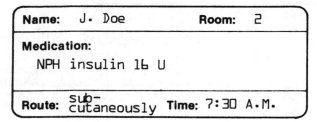

Name: J. Doe	**Room:** 2
Medication:	
NPH insulin 16 U	
Route: sub-cutaneously	**Time:** 7:30 A.M.

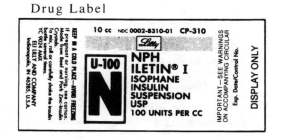

Indicate the correct dosage on the insulin syringe.

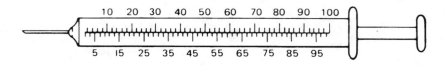

9. The physician has ordered 19 U of NPH U-100 insulin. Mark the correct dosage.

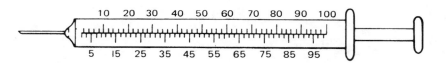

10. The physician has ordered heparin 4000 units. The drug label reads heparin 5000 units per milliliter. How many milliliters should the patient receive?

DRUGS IN POWDERED FORM

Some drugs are unstable in liquid form. They are packaged in powdered form in sterile ampules or vials and must be dissolved in a diluent, usually sterile normal saline or sterile distilled water, before they can be administered. Directions for dissolving powdered drugs will usually be found on the vial or on accompanying literature. These directions will generally state the type and amount of diluent to be used and the amount of drug per milliliter of solution. If no directions are available, it is common practice to dissolve the drug in the amount of diluent that will yield 1 to 2 ml containing the desired dose. When a single-dose vial is used, one adds 1 to 2 ml of diluent and withdraws the contents. Multiple-dose vials usually have a 10 to 20 ml capacity (indicated on the label); therefore, when contents of a multiple-dose vial are dissolved, the vial must be labeled with the amount of diluent used and the amount of drug per milliliter of solution.

Consider the following problem:

Drug Label

Name: J. Doe	Room: 3
Medication:	
Keflin 500 mg	
Route: I.M.	**Time:** q 6 h

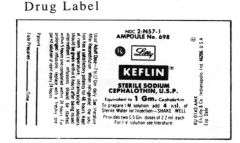

From the drug label, adding 4 ml of sterile water will yield enough solution for two doses. Each dose contains 0.5 g in 2.2 ml of solution.

The information on the drug label indicates

On hand

$$\frac{0.5 \text{ g}}{2.2 \text{ ml}}$$

From the drug order printout

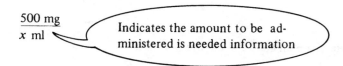

$$\frac{500 \text{ mg}}{x \text{ ml}}$$ Indicates the amount to be administered is needed information

The ratio from the order is set up using similar units in numerator and denominator. Since the units in the two numerators are not exactly the same, one of the units must be converted to the unit used in the other ratio.

In this case, change 0.5 g to milligrams:

$$0.5 \text{ g} = 500 \text{ mg}$$

The ratios are

Desired	On hand
$\dfrac{500 \text{ mg}}{x \text{ ml}}$	$\dfrac{500 \text{ mg}}{2.2 \text{ ml}}$

Replacing 0.5 g by 500 mg

Set the two ratios equal to form the proportion.

$$\frac{500 \text{ mg}}{x \text{ ml}} = \frac{500 \text{ mg}}{2.2 \text{ ml}}$$

Use the numerical data to determine the value of x:

$$\frac{500}{x} = \frac{500}{2.2}$$

$$500x = 500\,(2.2)$$

$$x = \frac{500\,(2.2)}{500}$$

$$x = 2.2$$

The correct answer is 2.2 ml.

EXAMPLE 4.3

Determine the correct dosage from the following.

Drug Label

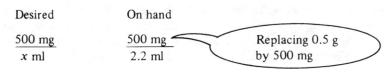

Name:	J. Doe	Room:	4

Medication:

   Prostaphlin 500 mg

Route:	I.M.	Time:	q 4 h

1. How much sterile water must be added to the vial? _____
2. Once the solution is constituted, 1.5 ml contains _____ mg of sodium ampicillin.
3. Use the information in step 2 to set up the drug-on-hand ratio.

$$\frac{\boxed{} \text{ mg}}{\boxed{} \text{ ml}}$$

4. Write a similar ratio for the drug desired:

$$\frac{\boxed{} \text{ mg}}{\boxed{} \text{ ml}}$$

5. Write a proportion using steps 3 and 4.

6. Solve for the unknown.

The order is for crystalline penicillin 400,000 U every 4 hours. The drug label reads crystalline penicillin 1,000,000 U in powder form. How many milliliters are necessary to produce a solution with 400,000 U?

When working with drugs in powder form and an order for a drug in units, the nurse chooses the amount of solution to administer to the patient. Once the nurse chooses the amount to be administered, the problem is to determine the amount of diluent to add to the powder to assure the proper concentration of solution. The nurse normally chooses 1 to 2 ml to be administered to the patient.

In the above problem, plan to administer 1 ml to the patient. Then the desired dosage is

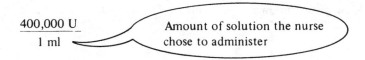

The on-hand information is

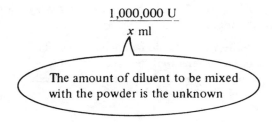

The number of milliliters to be mixed with the powder for a resulting solution containing 400,000 U/ml is the unknown. Set up the proportion

$$\frac{\text{Desired}}{400,000 \text{ U}} = \frac{\text{On hand}}{1,000,000 \text{ U}}$$
$$\frac{400,000 \text{ U}}{1 \text{ ml}} = \frac{1,000,000 \text{ U}}{x \text{ ml}}$$

Solve for x:

$$\frac{400,000}{1} = \frac{1,000,000}{x}$$
$$400,000x = 1,000,000 \, (1)$$
$$x = \frac{1,000,000}{400,000} = \frac{10}{4}$$
$$x = 2.5$$

Therefore 2.5 ml of diluent must be mixed with the powder.

Exercise 34

The following problems will give you practice with drugs in powdered form.

DIRECTIONS: Some of the following problems will require you to extract information from drug order printouts and drug labels. Compare the correct dosage for all problems. If a syringe is given, shade the syringe to indicate your answer.

1. The order is for Kefzol 500 mg IM bid. The drug label reads Kefzol equivalent to 1 g. Add 2.5 ml of sterile water for injection. Yields 3 ml reconstituted solution containing 330 mg/ml.

   How much sterile water should be added to the vial? _____
   What is the dosage strength of the prepared solution? _____
   How many milliliters should the patient receive? _____

2. The order is for ampicillin 250 mg IM every 4 hours. The drug label reads sodium ampicillin equivalent to 1 g. Add 3.4 ml of sterile water for injection to yield 4 ml reconstituted solution containing 250 mg/ml.

   How much sterile water should be added to the vial? _____
   What is the dosage strength of the prepared solution? _____
   How many milliliters should the patient receive? _____

   If the order reads ampicillin 150 mg every 4 hours, how many milliliters should the patient receive? _____

3. Drug Order Printout   Drug Label

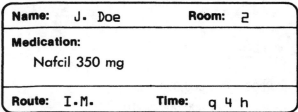

Name: J. Doe   **Room:** 2

Medication:
   Nafcil 350 mg

Route: I.M.   **Time:** q 4 h

How much sterile water should be added to the vial? _____
What is the dosage strength of the prepared solution? _____
How many milliliters should the patient receive? _____

4. Drug Order Printout

Name: J. Doe	**Room:** 2
Medication: Keflin 250 mg	
Route: I.M. **Time:** q 4 h	

Drug Label

NDC 2-N57-1
AMPOULE No. 698

KEFLIN®
STERILE SODIUM CEPHALOTHIN, U.S.P.
Equivalent to **1 Gm.** Cephalothin
To prepare I.M. solution add **4** m.l. of Sterile Water for Injection—SHAKE WELL
Provides two G 5 Gm. doses of 2.2 ml each
For I.V. solution see literature

How much sterile water should be added to the vial? _____
What is the dosage strength of the prepared solution? _____
How many milliliters should the patient receive? _____

5. The order is for streptomycin 500 mg every 6 hours. The drug label reads 5 g in 12.5 ml. How many milliliters should the patient receive? _____

6. The order is for Prostaphlin 500 mg every 8 hours. The drug label reads Prostaphlin 0.5 g. Add 2.7 ml of sterile water to yield 250 mg/1.5 ml.

How much sterile water should be added to the vial? _____
What is the dosage strength of the prepared solution? _____
How many milliliters should the patient receive? _____

7. Drug Order Printout

Name: J. Doe	**Room:** 2
Medication:	
Streptomycin 500 mg	
Route: I.M. **Time:** Every 4 h	

Drug Label

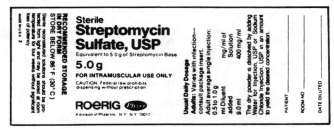

How much sterile water should be added to the vial? _____

What is the dosage strength of the prepared solution? _____

How many milliliters should the patient receive? _____

8. The order is for penicillin G 100,000 U IM every 6 hours. The drug label reads penicillin G 1,000,000 U. How many milliliters of sterile diluent are necessary to produce a solution with 100,000 U/ml?

9. The order is for staphcillin 500 mg every 6 hours. The drug label reads staphcillin equivalent to 1.0 g. Add 1.8 ml of sterile water for injection to yield 500 mg/ml.

How much sterile water should be added to the vial? _____

What is the dosage strength of the prepared solution? _____

How many milliliters should the patient receive? _____

10.   Drug Order Printout

Name: J. Doe		**Room:** 2
Medication:		
Geopen 1 g		
Route: I.M.	**Time:** q 6 h	

Drug Label

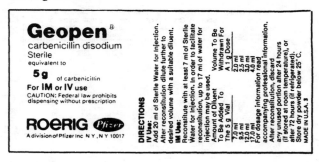

How much sterile water should be added to the vial? _____
What is the dosage strength of the prepared solution? _____
How many milliliters should the patient receive? _____

11.   The order is for streptomycin 500 mg IM every 6 hours. The drug label reads streptomycin equivalent to 5 g. How many milliliters of sterile diluent are necessary to produce a solution with 500 mg/ml?

12. The order is for Claforan 1 g IV every 8 hours. How many milliliters of sterile diluent are necessary to produce a solution with 1 g?

PREPARATION OF CLAFORAN STERILE

Claforan for IM or IV administration should be reconstituted as follows:

Strength	Diluent (mL)	Withdrawable Volume (mL)	Approximate Concentration (mg/mL)
1g vial (IM)*	3	3 4	300
2g vial (IM)*	5	6 0	330
1g vial (IV)*	10	10 4	95
2g vial (IV)*	10	11 0	180
1g infusion	50-100	50-100	20-10
2g infusion	50-100	50-100	40-20
10g bottle	47	52 0	200
10g bottle	97	102 0	100

*in conventional vials

Shake to dissolve; inspect for particulate matter and discoloration prior to use Solutions of Claforan range from very pale yellow to light amber, depending on concentration, diluent used, and length and condition of storage.

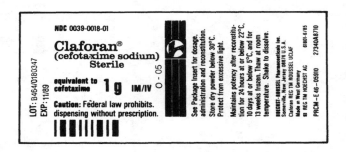

13. The order is for Chloromycetin 500 mg IM every 4 hours. How many milliliters of sterile diluent are necessary to produce a solution with 1 g?

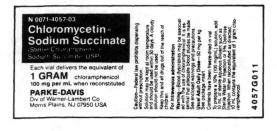

14. The order is for Keflin 250 mg. The drug label reads Keflin provides two 0.5 g doses of 2.2 ml each. How many milliliters does the patient receive?

15. The order is for Prostaphlin 150 mg. The drug label reads Prostaphlin equivalent to 1 g. Add 5.7 milliliters sterile water for injection. Each 1.5 ml contains 250 mg. How many milliliters does the patient receive?

ANSWERS TO EXAMPLES

Example 4.1

1. 100 mg/2 ml
2. 25 mg
3. On hand   Desired

$$\frac{2 \text{ ml}}{100 \text{ mg}} \qquad \frac{x \text{ ml}}{25 \text{ mg}}$$

$$\frac{2}{100} = \frac{x}{25}$$

$$100x = 2(25)$$

$$100x = 50$$

$$x = \frac{50}{100}$$

$$x = 0.5 \text{ or } \frac{1}{2}$$

correct dosage $\frac{1}{2}$ ml

Example 4.2

1. 1000 mg/2 ml
2. 500 mg
3. On hand   Desired

$$\frac{2 \text{ ml}}{1000 \text{ mg}} \qquad \frac{x \text{ ml}}{500 \text{ mg}}$$

$$\frac{2}{1000} = \frac{x}{500}$$

$$1000x = 1000$$

$$x = \frac{1000}{1000} = 1$$

1 ml is correct dosage

4.

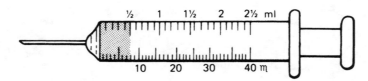

Example 4.3

1. 2.7 ml

2. 1.5 ml contains 250 mg;

3. On hand

$$\frac{250 \text{ mg}}{1.5 \text{ ml}}$$

5. $\dfrac{500 \text{ mg}}{x \text{ ml}} = \dfrac{250 \text{ mg}}{1.5 \text{ ml}}$

6. $\dfrac{500}{x} = \dfrac{250}{1.5}$

$$250x = 750.0$$

$$x = \frac{750}{250} = 3$$

$$x = 3$$

3 ml is correct dosage.

The directions on the drug label specify the exact amount of sterile water.
Drug label specifies the amount of solution yielded by adding sterile water.
250 ml is contained in each 1.5 ml

4. Desired

$$\frac{500 \text{ mg}}{x \text{ ml}}$$

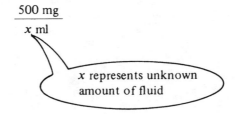

x represents unknown amount of fluid

5 INTRAVENOUS MEDICATIONS

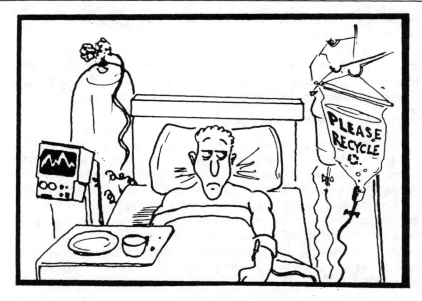

CHAPTER OBJECTIVES

- Demonstrate proficiency when calculating the intravenous infusion rates with varying drop factor sets
- Determine the correct length of time for intravenous infusions
- Calculate the correct flow rates for intravenous piggyback medications

INTRODUCTION

This chapter focuses on the nurse's responsibility for adminstering intravenous fluids and medications. The two major areas of responsibility include the administration of intravenous fluids in large volumes (such as 1000 milliliters of dextrose in water) and the administration of intravenous piggybacks with small volumes of solution. These small volumes usually are 50 or 100 milliliters containing medications for intravenous infusion.

The nurse must be familiar with the drop factor of each intravenous set up. The drop factor refers to the size of each drop and the number of drops necessary to deliver one milliliter of solution. For example, some equipment yields 1 milliliter after 10 drops, while on other equipment 15 drops yields 1 milliliter; still other sets yield 1 milliliter after 60 drops. It is the nurse's responsibility to check drop factors on all equipment sets and correctly calculate infusion rates based on the drop factor.

To better understand the influence of the drop factor, look at the following situations. Consider an IV set up where the nurse adjusts the infusion rate to 20 drops per minute and runs the IV for 2 hours.

20 drops per minute yields
20 × 60 drops in 60 minutes,
1200 drops in 1 hour, so
2400 drops in 2 hours.

Now consider the effect of the drop factor in three situations:

Situation	Drop factor in gtt/ml	For 2400 drops in 2 hours the total volume infused
1	10 gtt/ml	2400/10 or 240 ml
2	15 gtt/ml	2400/15 or 160 ml
3	60 gtt/ml	2400/60 or 40 ml

As one can see, the drop factor significantly influences the total volume infused over a fixed period of time at a fixed rate.

The drop factor of intravenous equipment is a fixed value (specific to that piece of equipment) and will appear on the instruction of the equipment. The nurse must calculate the infusion rate if the time and volume are given or must calculate the time of infusion if the rate and volume are given. Each of the following sections deals with these aspects of intravenous administration.

DETERMINING INTRAVENOUS INFUSION RATES

This section focuses on the nurse's responsibility for administering intravenous fluids in large volumes. The intravenous route of administering fluids allows for the fastest absorption as the fluids are injected directly into the patient's circulatory system via selected veins. Intravenous fluids are often given to the patient to correct electrolyte imbalances or to treat various disorders or diseases.

The physician ordering intravenous fluids specifies the total volume, the type of solution, and the total infusion time. To deliver the requested volume in the time specified by the physician, it is the nurse's responsibility to calculate the proper rate of flow. All intravenous administration sets are calibrated in *drops per milliliter (gtt/ml)*. It is important that the nurse check the type of intravenous set used, as different manufacturers produce intravenous sets that yield a varying number of drops per milliliter.

The following formula will assist the nurse in determining the number of drops per minute to administer intravenous fluids correctly.

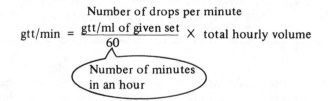

$$\text{gtt/min} = \frac{\text{gtt/ml of given set}}{60} \times \text{total hourly volume}$$

Number of drops per minute

Number of minutes in an hour

Use the formula to determine the correct drops per minute for the following problem. The physician has ordered 50 ml 5% dextrose in water with 50 mg ampicillin per hour. The set available yields 10 gtt/ml. The nurse must determine the number of drops per minute the intravenous should infuse. Referring to the formula and the physician's order, we have

gtt/ml of given set = 10

Total hourly volume = 50 ml

Substitute in the formula:

$$\text{gtt/min} = \frac{10}{60} \times 50 = \frac{500}{60} = 8.33$$

Regulate the infusion to 8 drops per minute.

EXAMPLE 5.1*

The physician orders 100 ml 5% dextrose in water with 25 mg ampicillin per hour. Set yields 15 gtt/ml.

1. gtt per ml given set = _____ .
2. Total hourly volume = _____ .
3. Substitute in the formula.

4. Determine the drops per minute.

Often the information is not in a form allowing direct substitution in the formula. Usually the rate is not given. In these cases you must calculate the rate at which the intravenous is to drip. Consider this problem. If 1000 ml of isotonic saline is to run over a period of 12 hours, how many drops are needed to regulate the flow (10 gtt/ml)?

Because the hourly rate is not given, you must determine the hourly rate before proceeding as in Example 4.6. Notice 1000 ml is to be given over 12 hours, so

$$\frac{1000 \text{ ml}}{12 \text{ h}}$$

will tell us the number of milliliters to be given each hour. Dividing 12 into 1000 yields

$$
\begin{array}{r}
83.33 \\
12{\overline{\smash{\big)}\,1000.0}} \\
\underline{96} \\
40 \\
\underline{36} \\
40 \\
\underline{36} \\
40 \\
\underline{36} \\
4
\end{array}
$$

Thus 83.33 ml/hr. Substitute the values in the formula:

$$gtt/min = \frac{10}{60} \times 83.33$$

$$= \frac{1\cancel{0}}{6\cancel{0}} \times 83.33$$

$$= \frac{83.33}{6} = 13.89$$

The infusion should be regulated to 14 drops per minute.

*Answers to the examples appear on page 142.

EXAMPLE 5.2

The physician orders 1000 ml 5% dextrose in water to run for 8 hours (10 gtt/ml set).

1. What is the total hourly volume?
2. gtt/ml of the given set = _____ .
3. Substitute in the formula.

4. Determine the drops per minute.

Exercise 35

For practice with intravenous fluids, solve the following problems.

1. The physician has ordered 500 ml of 5% dextrose in water to run over a period of 12 hours. How many drops per minute should the IV infuse (10 gtt/ml set)?

2. The physician has ordered 1000 ml of dextrose in water to run over a 12-hour period. How many drops per minute should the IV infuse (10 gtt/ml set)?

3. The physician orders 2000 ml 5% dextrose in water over a 24-hour period. How many drops per minute should the IV infuse (15 gtt/ml set)?

4. The order is for 1000 ml of 5% dextrose in water to run at 250 ml/hour. How many drops per minute should the IV infuse (20 gtt/ml set)?

5. Administer 1000 ml isotonic saline in 4 hours. How many drops per minute should the IV infuse (10 gtt/ml set)?

6. The physician orders 500 ml of 5% dextrose in water over an 8-hour period. How many drops per minute should the IV infuse (10 gtt/ml set)?

7. The order is for 500 ml of 5% dextrose in water to be administered in 4 hours. How many drops per minute should the IV infuse (15 gtt/ml set)?

8. The physician orders 3000 ml 5% dextrose in water to run over a 24-hour period. How many drops per minute should the IV infuse (10 gtt/ml set)?

9. The physician orders 500 ml to run at 250 ml per hour. How many drops per minute should the IV infuse (10 gtt/ml set)?

LENGTH OF TIME FOR INTRAVENOUS INFUSIONS

Often a physician will order an intravenous infusion and specify the rate at which the IV is to be administered. To maintain an IV schedule for each individual patient, it is necessary that the nurse be able to calculate the number of hours the infusion should last.

The nurse should use the formula:

$$\text{number of gtt/min} = \frac{\text{number of ml ordered}}{\text{number of min the IV is to infuse}} \times \text{drop factor}$$

For example, the physician orders 1200 ml of normal saline to infuse at 50 gtt/min. The drop factor is 15 gtt/min. How many hours must the IV run?

Substituting:

$$50 = \frac{1200}{x}(15)$$

$$50x = 1200(15)$$

$$50x = 18000$$

$$x = \frac{18000}{50}$$

$$x = 360$$

This is the number of minutes, thus

$$\text{Hours} = \frac{x}{60} = \frac{360}{60} = 6$$

$$\text{Hours} = 6.$$

EXAMPLE 5.3

The physician orders 1000 ml of 5% dextrose in water to infuse at 40 gtt/min. How many hours must the IV infuse? (10 gtt/ml set)

1. What are the drops per minute requested?

2. What are the drops per milliliter of the given set?

3. How many milliliters were ordered?

4. Substitute in the formula to determine the number of minutes for the IV to infuse.

5. What is the number of hours?

Exercise 36

Calculate the time of infusion.

1. The physician orders 100 ml Ringers lactate to infuse at 20 gtt/min. How many hours must the IV infuse? (60 gtt/ml set)

2. The physician orders 1200 ml of normal saline to infuse at 50 gtt/min. How many hours must the IV infuse? (10 gtt/ml set)

3. The physician orders 1000 ml of 10% glucose to infuse at 35 gtt/min. How many hours must the IV infuse? (15 gtt/ml set)

4. The physician orders 900 ml of 5% dextrose in water to infuse at 40 gtt/min. How many hours must the IV infuse? (10 gtt/ml set)

5. The physician orders 1500 ml Ringers lactate to infuse at 45 gtt/min. How many hours must the IV infuse? (10 gtt/ml set)

6. The physician orders 100 ml of 5% dextrose in water to infuse at 30 gtt/min. How many hours must the IV infuse? (60 gtt/ml set)

7. The physician orders 800 ml physiologic saline to infuse at 50 gtt/min. How many hours must the IV infuse? (10 gtt/ml set)

8. The physician orders 500 ml of Ringers lactate to infuse at 40 gtt/min. How many hours must the IV infuse? (60 gtt/ml set)

9. The physician orders 200 ml of 5% glucose to infuse at 50 gtt/min. How many hours must the IV infuse? (60 gtt/ml set)

INTRAVENOUS PIGGYBACK MEDICATIONS

This section focuses on the nurse's responsibility for intravenous piggyback infusions. The piggyback intravenous medication is connected to a primary infusion set up and is ordered specifically for the purpose of delivering a variety of medications to a patient. The patient is usually already receiving intravenous fluids from a primary intravenous set up. The piggyback is attached via a needle to an adaptor on the existing primary tubing.

Intravenous piggyback (IVPB) medications are usually dissolved in 50 ml or 100 ml of dextrose in water or physiologic saline and are infused in 30 to 60 minutes. In many hospitals the pharmacy is responsible for preparing piggyback medications, and they are delivered to nursing units ready for administration. It is common practice for nurses to be responsible for administering numerous IVPB medications during a daily work experience.

Before administering IVPB medications, it is necessary to calculate the flow rate or drops per minute to deliver the 50 ml or 100 ml of solution in 30 to 60 minutes. To do this the nurse must first determine the drop factor of the equipment selected to infuse the IVPB. The drop factor (10 gtt/ml, 15 gtt/ml, or 60 gtt/ml) is usually indicated on the equipment selected to administer the infusion.

Nurses are always responsible for checking administration time for all intravenous medications in appropriate references. Intervals of 30 and 60 minutes have been arbitrarily chosen because these are commonly used infusion times for most IVPB medications.

The following formula will assist the nurse in determining the number of drops per minute to administer intravenous fluids piggyback.

Numbers of drops per minute for piggybacks

$$\frac{\text{number}}{\text{of}} = \frac{\text{number of ml ordered}}{\text{number of min the IV}} \times \frac{\text{drop}}{\text{factor}}$$
$$\text{gtt/min} \qquad\qquad \text{is to infuse}$$

EXAMPLE 5.4

Consider the following order:

        Keflin 2 g IVPB q 6 hr

        Infuse in 1 hour

The piggyback label reads:

        Keflin 2 g in 100 ml 5% dextrose in water

        (60 gtt/ml set)

1. gtt per ml of given set = _____ .
2. Total time in minutes = _____ .
3. gtt per min = _____ .
4. Total milliliters ordered = _____ .
5. Substitute in the formula.

6. Determine the drops per minute.

Exercise 37

For practice with IV piggybacks, solve the following problems.

1. The physician has ordered Nebcin 60 mg IVPB. The IVPB label reads Nebcin 60 mg in 50 milliliters normal saline. The drop factor is 10 gtt/ml. Infuse in thirty minutes. How many drops per minute should the IVPB infuse?

2. The physician has ordered ampicillin 250 mg IVPB. The IVPB label reads ampicillin 250 mg in 100 milliliters 5% dextrose in water. The drop factor is 15 gtt/ml. Infuse in thirty minutes. How many drops per minute should the IVPB infuse?

3. The order is for Tagamet 300 mg IVPB. The IVPB label reads Tagamet 300 mg in 100 milliliters 5% dextrose in water. The drop factor is 60 gtt/ml. Infuse in one hour. How many drops per minute should the IVPB infuse?

4. The order is for gentamicin 50 mg IVPB. The IVPB label reads gentamicin 50 mg in 50 milliliters physiologic saline. The drop factor is 60 gtt/ml. Infuse in thirty minutes. How many drops per minute should the IVPB infuse?

5. The physician has ordered Ancef 1 g IVPB. The IVPB label reads Ancef 1 g in 50 milliliters physiologic saline. The drop factor is 10 gtt/ml. Infuse in thirty minutes. How many drops per minute should the IVPB infuse?

6. The physician has ordered Mefoxin 1 g IVPB. The IVPB label reads Mefoxin 1 g in 100 milliliters physiologic saline. The drop factor is 15 gtt/ml. Infuse in one hour. How many drops per minute should the IVPB infuse?

7. The order is for ampicillin 1 g IVPB. The IVPB label reads ampicillin 1 g in 100 milliliters of 5% dextrose in water. The drop factor is 60 gtt/ml. Infuse in one hour. How many drops per minute should the IVPB infuse?

8. The physician has ordered Cefabid 2 g IVPB. The IVPB label reads Cefabid 2 g in 100 milliliters physiologic saline. The drop factor is 10 gtt/ml. Infuse in thirty minutes. How many drops per minute should the IVPB infuse?

9. The order is for gentamicin 50 mg IVPB. The IVPB label reads gentamicin 50 mg in 100 milliliters 5% dextrose in water. The drop factor is 15 gtt/ml. Infuse in one hour. How many drops per minute should the IVPB infuse?

ANSWERS TO EXAMPLES

Example 5.1

1. 15
2. 100 ml
3. $\text{gtt/min} = \frac{15}{60} \times 100$
4. $\frac{15}{60} \times 100 = \frac{150\cancel{0}}{6\cancel{0}} = 25$

   25 gtt/min

Example 5.2

1. 1000 ml to run for 8 hours. Divide 8 into 1000 to get the milliliters per hour:

$$
\begin{array}{r}
125. \\
8\overline{)1000.} \qquad \text{Result 125 ml/hour} \\
\underline{8} \\
20 \\
\underline{16} \\
40 \\
\underline{40} \\
0
\end{array}
$$

2. gtt/ml = 10
3. $\text{gtt/min} = \frac{10}{60} \times 125$
4. $\frac{10}{60} \times 125 = \frac{1}{6} \times 125 = \frac{125}{6} = 20.83$

   Round off to 21

   Adjust infusion to 21 gtt/min

Example 5.3

1. 40 gtt/min
2. 10 gtt/ml
3. 1000 ml
4. $40 = \frac{1000(10)}{x}$

   $40x = 1000(10)$

   $x = \frac{10000}{40}$

   $x = 250$ minutes

5. Hours $= \frac{250}{60} = 4$ hours 10 minutes

Example 5.4

1. 60 gtt/ml
2. 60 minutes
3. x, the unknown
4. 100 ml
5. $x = \frac{100}{60} (60)$
6. $x = \frac{100}{60} (60)$

   $x = 100$ gtt/min

6 PEDIATRIC MEDICATIONS

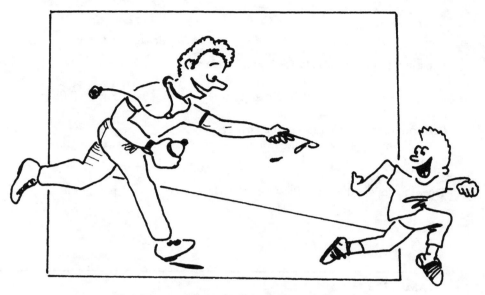

But Timmy, this stuff will make you feel better!

CHAPTER OBJECTIVES

- Calculate the correct pediatric dosage using weight in kilograms as well as various pediatric rules
- Determine the correct pediatric dosage when applying the surface-area formula

INTRODUCTION

Many hospitals have special divisions for infants and children; sometimes infants and children are integrated with adult patients throughout the hospital. The child should not be considered a miniature adult but a unique individual who requires approaches and treatments different from those of adults.

This chapter focuses specifically on the calculation of dosage for infants and children. Infants and children always require smaller quantities of medications than adults; therefore it is important that nurses caring for children know the safe range of dosages. The physician will always prescribe medications, but nurses must be aware of usual dosage for frequently administered medications so that an overdose will not be given.

RULES

Young's Rule

Several rules have been formulated to serve as a guide for estimating the correct dosage for infants and children. One of these is Young's rule, designed for children from ages 1 or 2 years to 12 years.

Young's rule (1 or 2 years to 12 years of age):

$$\text{Child's dose} = \frac{\text{child age in years}}{\text{child age in years} + 12} \times \text{adult dose}$$

To determine how much aspirin a 3-year-old child should receive if the adult dose is 0.3 g, use Young's rule. The information needed is

$$\text{Child's age in years} = 3$$

$$\text{Child's age in years} + 12 = 15$$

$$\text{Adult dosage} = 0.3 \text{ g}$$

Substituting in the formula for Young's rule yields

$$\text{Child's dose} = \frac{3}{15} \times 0.3 \text{ g} = \frac{0.9}{15} \text{ g} = 0.06 \text{ g}$$

Performing the division gives the answer as 0.06 g.

Aspirin is usually measured in grains, so change the answer to grains:

$$0.06 \text{ g} = 1 \text{ gr}$$

Thus the child's dose is 0.06 g = gr i. The correct dosage is 1 grain.

EXAMPLE 6.1*

How much Demerol should a 6-year-old child receive if the adult dose is 75 mg? Use young's rule.

1. Child's age in years = _____ .
2. Child's age in years + 12 = _____ .
3. Adult dose = _____ .
4. Substitute the values in Young's rule.

5. Solve for the child's dosage.

EXAMPLE 6.2

How much atropine sulfate should a 4-year-old child receive if the average adult dose is gr $\frac{1}{150}$? Use Young's rule.

1. Child's age in years = _____ .
2. Child's age in years + 12 = _____ .
3. Adult dose = _____ .
4. Substitute the values in Young's rule.

5. Solve for the child's dose.

Fried's Rule

The second rule, Fried's rule, is designed for computing dosage for infants. Fried's rule is designed for infants from birth to 1 or 2 years of age.

Fried's rule (birth to 1 or 2 years of age):

$$\text{Infant's dose} = \frac{\text{age in months}}{150} \times \text{adult dose}$$

The physician orders codeine for a 10-month-old infant. If the adult dose is gr $\frac{1}{2}$, how much codeine should the infant receive? Since the infant is less than 2 years old, apply Fried's rule.

The child's age in months is 10.

The adult dose is gr $\frac{1}{2}$.

$$\text{Infant's dose} = \frac{10}{150} \times \frac{1}{2}$$

$$= \frac{1\cancel{0}}{15\cancel{0}} \times \frac{1}{2} = \frac{1}{15 \times 2} = \frac{1}{30}$$

Infant dose is gr $\frac{1}{30}$.

EXAMPLE 6.3

Find the dosage of Nembutal for a 6-month-old infant if the adult dose is 90 mg.
  To apply Fried's rule determine:

1. Age of infant in months = _____ .
2. Adult dose = _____ .
3. Substitute the value in Fried's rule.

4. Solve for infant dosage.

EXAMPLE 6.4

If an adult receives 300 mg of Ilosone, what is the correct dosage for an 18-month-old infant?

1. Age of infant in months = _____ .
2. Adult dose = _____ .
3. Substitute values in Fried's rule.

4. Solve for infant dosage.

Clark's Rule

The third rule, Clark's rule, uses the weight of the child and the weight of an average adult. Therefore it can be used to determine the dosage for infants and children, regardless of age. Clark's rule provides more accurate information than either Fried's or Young's rule.

Clark's rule (all ages):

$$\text{Child's dose} = \frac{\text{weight of child in pounds}}{150 \text{ lb}} \times \text{adult dose}$$

The 150 pounds in Clark's rule is the average weight of an adult.

How much phenobarbital should a 70-pound child receive if the adult dosage is 60 mg?

Child's weight = 70

Adult dosage = 60 mg

Substituting these values in Clark's rule gives

$$\text{Child's dose} = \frac{70}{150} \times 60 \text{ mg}$$

Solving for the child's dose, we have

$$\frac{70}{150} \times 60 = \frac{420}{15} = 28 \text{ mg}$$

Child's dose = 28 mg.

EXAMPLE 6.5

An adult receives aspirin gr x. How many grains of aspirin should be given to a child weighing 45 lbs?

1. Weight of child in pounds = _____ .
2. Adult dose = _____ .
3. Substitute the values in the formula for Clark's rule.

4. Solve for the child's dose.

EXAMPLE 6.6

An adult receives aspirin gr x. How many grains of aspirin should be given to a child weighing 60 lbs?

1. Weight of child in pounds = _____ .
2. Adult dose = _____ .

3. Solve for the child's dosage using Clark's rule.

Surface-Area Rule

The fourth rule for determining children's drug dosage, the surface-area method, uses the surface area of the infant in computing the dosage. The surface area is measured in square meters (m^2), and a nomogram must be consulted to determine the body surface area. If the nomogram is available, this method provides the most accurate determination of the correct children's dosage.

Surface-area rule

$$\text{Child's dose} = \frac{\text{Surface area of child in square meters}}{1.7 \text{ m}^2} \times \text{adult dose}$$

The accepted average adult surface area is 1.7 m^2.

The physician orders Keflin for a child. The adult dosage for Keflin is 100 mg. What is the dosage for a child with a surface area of 1.2 m^2?

Using the surface-area formula

$$\text{Child's dose} = \frac{1.2 \text{ m}^2}{1.7 \text{ m}^2} \times 100 \text{ mg}$$

$$\text{Child's dose} = \frac{120}{1.7} = 70.6 = 71 \text{ mg}$$

The correct dosage for the child is 71 mg.

EXAMPLE 6.7

The adult dose for Demerol is 50 mg. A child with a surface area of 0.30 m^2 should receive how much Demerol?

1. Surface area of child in square meters = _____ .
2. Adult dose = _____ .
3. Substitute the values in the surface-area formula.

4. Solve for the child's dosage.

Exercise 38

Find the correct child's dosage.

1. The adult dose of phenobarbital is 60 mg. How much should a 6-year-old receive?

2. The adult dose of morphine sulfate is 12 mg. How much should a 6-year-old receive?

3. The daily dose of Dilantin is 30 to 100 mg for an adult. Compute the dosage for a child weighing 35 lb using *(a)* the minimum adult dose and *(b)* the maximum adult dose.

4. The adult dose of aspirin is gr *x*. How many grains should be given to a child who weighs 20 lb?

5. The adult dose of codeine sulfate is 30 mg. What is the dose for a 20-month-old infant?

6. The adult dose of Demerol is 50 to 100 mg. Compute the dosage for a 6-month-old infant using *(a)* the minimum adult dose and *(b)* the maximum adult dose.

7. The adult dose for Garamycin is 80 mg. How much Garamycin would a child of 4 years receive?

8. The adult dose for Demerol is 75 mg. How much Demerol would a 3-year-old child receive?

9. The adult dose for streptomycin is 500 mg. How much streptomycin would a 3-year-old child receive?

10. The adult dose for tetracycline is 500 mg. How much tetracycline would a child of 7 years receive?

11. The adult dose for penicillin is 600,000 U. How much should a 3-year-old child receive?

12. The adult dose for Gantrisin is 1000 mg. What should be the dose for a 10-month-old infant?

13. The adult dose for Demerol is 50 mg. How much Demerol would a 9-month-old infant receive?

14. The adult dose for morphine is 12 mg. How much morphine should a 6-month-old infant receive?

15. The adult dose for ampicillin is 500 mg. How much ampicillin should a 12-month-old infant receive?

16. The adult dose of adrenalin is 1 mg. What is the dose of adrenalin for a child weighing 40 lb?

17. The adult dose of sodium luminal is 100 mg. What is the dose of sodium luminal for a child weighing 25 lb?

18. The adult dose of Keflin is 100 mg. What is the dose of Keflin for an infant weighing 10 lb?

19. The adult dose of Kefzol is 500 mg. What is the dose of Kefzol for an infant weighing 20 lb?

20. The adult dose of atropine is gr $\frac{1}{150}$. What is the dose for an infant with a body surface area of 0.44 m²?

21. The adult dose of Keflin is 250 mg. What is the dose of Keflin for an infant with a body surface area of 0.45 m²?

22. The adult dose of Demerol is 50 mg. What is the dose of Demerol for an infant with a body surface area of 0.22 m²?

23. The adult dose of Garamycin is 60 mg. How much Garamycin should an infant with a body surface area of 0.40 m² receive?

CALCULATING DOSAGE PER KILOGRAM OF BODY WEIGHT

Another very accurate method of calculating pediatric medications uses the child's weight in kilograms. A two-step process is used to calculate the child's dosage. First, calculate 24-hour dosage. Second, calculate the dosage for each administration using the 24-hour dosage information.

1. Child's 24-hour dosage $= \left(\dfrac{\text{medication dosage per}}{\text{kilogram body weight}} \times \dfrac{\text{child's weight}}{\text{in kilograms}} \right)$

2. Child's dosage $= \dfrac{\text{(child's 24-hour dosage)} \times \text{(hours between administration)}}{24}$

Consider the problem:
The physician orders kanamycin sulfate IM q 12 hours.
The drug label reads: kanamycin sulfate 75 mg/2 ml.
Normal pediatric dosage is: 15 mg/kg/day.
How much kanamycin should a child weighing 10 kg be given?
From what is given, we know:
    medication dosage per kilogram body weight = 15 mg/kg/day
    child's weight in kilograms = 10 kg
    hours between medication administrations = 12 hrs
1. Child's 24-hour dosage = 15 × 10 = 150 mg,
    thus 150 mg of kanamycin in 24-hour period
2. Child's dosage $= \dfrac{150 \times 12}{24} = 75$ mg

Thus the child is to receive 75 mg per dose.

EXAMPLE 6.8

The physician orders Pyopen IM q 6 hours. The drug label reads Pyopen 1 g/2.5 ml and the normal pediatric dosage is 100 mg/kg/day. How much Pyopen should a child weighing 20 kg be given?

1. What is the medication dosage per kilogram body weight?
2. What is the child's weight in kilograms?
3. How many hours between medication administrations?

ANSWERS TO EXAMPLES

Example 6.1

1. 6
2. 18, adding 12 to child's age (6) = 18.
3. 75 mg
4. Child's dose $= \frac{6}{18} \times 75$

5.
$$
\begin{array}{r}
75 \\
\times 6 \\
\hline
450
\end{array}
$$

$$
\begin{array}{r}
25 \\
18\overline{)450} \\
36 \\
\hline
90 \\
90 \\
\hline
0
\end{array}
$$

Short Method

$$\overset{1}{\underset{3}{\cancel{\frac{6}{18}}}} \times 75 = \frac{75}{3} = 25$$

Child's dose = 25 mg

Example 6.2

1. 4.
2. 16; 4 + 12 = 16
3. gr $\frac{1}{150}$
4. Child's dose $= \frac{4}{16} \times \frac{1}{150}$

5. $\frac{4}{16} \times \frac{1}{150} = \overset{1}{\underset{4}{\cancel{\frac{4}{16}}}} \times \frac{1}{150} = \frac{1}{600}$

gr $\frac{1}{600}$

Example 6.3

1. 6
2. 90 mg
3. Infant dosage $= \frac{6}{150} \times 90$
4. Infant dosage $= \frac{6}{150} \times 90 = \frac{540}{150} = 3.6$ mg

4 mg is the correct dosage.

Example 6.4

1. 18
2. 300 mg
3. Infant's dosage $= \frac{18}{150} \times 300$ mg
4. Infant's dosage $= \underset{1}{\cancel{\frac{18}{150}}} \times \overset{2}{\cancel{300}} = 18 \times 2 = 36$ mg

Example 6.5

1. 45
2. 10 gr
3. Child's dose $= \frac{45}{150} \times 10$ gr
4. Child's dose $= \frac{45}{\underset{15}{150}} \times \overset{1}{\cancel{10}} = \frac{45}{15} = 3$

   3 gr is the child's dosage.

Example 6.6

1. 60
2. 10 gr
3. Child's dose $= \frac{60}{150} \times 10$

   $= \frac{\cancel{60}}{\cancel{150}} \times 10$

   $= \frac{60}{15} \times 4$

   Child's dose $= 4$ gr

Example 6.7

1. 0.30
2. 50 mg
3. Child's dose $= \frac{0.30}{1.7} \times 50$
4. Child's dose $= \frac{0.30 \times 50}{1.7}$

   $= \frac{15}{1.7} = 8.8$ mg

   Child's dose $= 9$ mg

Example 6.8

1. 100 mg/kg/day
2. 20 kg
3. 6 hours
4. $100(20) = 2000$
5. $\frac{2000(6)}{24} = \frac{2000}{4} = 500$ mg

7 PREPARATION OF SOLUTIONS

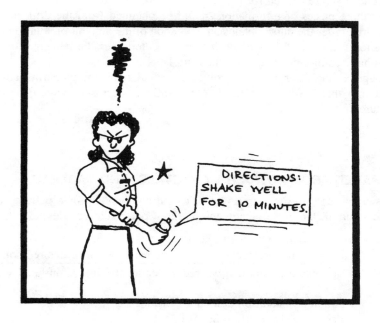

CHAPTER OBJECTIVES

- Calculate solutions prepared from powders, crystals, or tablets
- Demonstrate proficiency when computing solutions prepared from liquid solutes
- Exhibit proficiency calculating solutions prepared from solutes with concentrations other than 100 percent concentration

INTRODUCTION

Most hospital pharmacies have stock supplies of the most common solutions, which are readily available upon request. However, in smaller hospitals or in rural areas it may become the nurse's responsibility to prepare solutions of varying strengths for patient treatments. Solutions are most often used as disinfectants, for soaks, irrigations, mouthwashes, and other topical applications.

Solutions are prepared from drugs obtained in three different forms. First, the drug may be a solid such as powders, tablets, or crystals. Powders, tablets, and crystals are usually pure drugs; that is, the contents are considered 100 percent drug. Second, the drug may be a liquid and pure drug (once again, 100 percent drug). Third, the drug may be in liquid form but have a concentration that is less than 100 percent pure. The drug label will indicate when a drug is of a concentration that is less than 100 percent by stating the concentration, such as

> 50% alcohol solution

If the drug label does not indicate the concentration, it is assumed that the drug is 100 percent pure. A single mathematical formula is involved in calculations for preparing solutions. The formula is

$$\frac{\text{amount of solute needed for preparation}}{\text{amount of solution desired}} = \frac{\text{concentration of desired solution}}{\text{concentration of on-hand solute}}$$

The amount of solute needed for preparation is what the nurse must calculate to prepare a solution. The other three pieces of information should be obtained from the drug order and the drug label. From the drug order the nurse obtains an indication of the amount of solution desired and the percent concentration wanted in the solution. The nurse determines the percent concentration of the solute (drug) on hand using information on the drug label.

Although a single formula is involved in calculations for preparing solutions, this chapter is separated into three sections, reflecting the different forms in which the solutes (or drugs) are manufactured.

SOLUTIONS PREPARED FROM POWDERS, CRYSTALS, AND TABLETS

The physician orders sterile warm 5% boric acid compresses for a patient. To prepare 1000 ml of boric acid solution, the nurse obtains the bottle of boric acid crystals. Use the formula

$$\frac{\text{amount of solute needed for preparation}}{\text{amount of solution desired}} = \frac{\text{concentration of desired solution}}{\text{concentration of on-hand solute}}$$

Amount of solution desired = 1000
Percentage concentration of desired solution = 5
Percentage concentration of on-hand solute = 100

Recall pure drugs are 100%

Amount of solute needed for preparation of solution = x g

Crystals are measured in grams

Substituting in the formula gives

$$\frac{x}{1000} = \frac{5}{100}$$

Solving, we get

$$\frac{x}{1000} = \frac{5}{100}$$

$$100x = 5000$$

$$x = \frac{5000}{100} = 50$$

Therefore 50 g of boric acid crystals is added to 1000 ml of sterile water to prepare the solution.

When dealing with solutes in solid form, the nurse mixes the powder or crystals with about half the total volume of sterile water and stirs until the crystals dissolve or the mixture becomes saturated. The nurse then adds more sterile water and dilutes the mixture until the desired volume of solution is obtained. Because the volume of sterile water varies with the type of powder or crystals used, we will merely specify that the nurse is to dilute to the desired volume.

When using the formula with solutes in solid form, use the weight measure from the same system used to express the desired amount of solution. If milliliters are wanted, measure the solute in grams; if minims are wanted, measure the solute in grains.

EXAMPLE 7.1*

Prepare 2 oz of 8% iodine solution (from iodine crystals).

1. Amount of solution desired = _____ .
2. Concentration of desired solution = _____ .
3. Concentration of on-hand solute = _____ .
4. Solve for the amount of solute needed to prepare the solution.

Frequently the solute is obtained in tablet form. The next example involves such a solute.

EXAMPLE 7.2

Prepare 30 ml of a 10% sodium bicarbonate solution.

1. Amount of solution desired = _____ .
2. Concentration of desired solution = _____ .
3. Concentration of on-hand solute = _____ .
4. Solve for the amount of solute needed to prepare the solution.

5. If each tablet contains 10 grains of sodium bicarbonate, how many tablets are used?

SOLUTIONS PREPARED FROM PURE LIQUID SOLUTES

In working with pure liquid solutes, the amount of solute is determined using the same mathematical formula as in the previous section. The difference in working with liquid and solid solutes is the characteristics of the solutes. When sodium chloride solute (table salt) is added to sterile water and mixed, the salt dissolves, but more importantly the volume of water does not appreciably increase.

---

*Answers to examples appear on pages 166-167.

On the other hand, when a liquid solute such as 10 ml of fluid is added to 100 ml of water, the result is 110 ml of solution. Thus if it is determined (by using the formula) that 10 ml of solute is added, then the amount of solute is subtracted from the desired volume. The difference is the amount of sterile water to be used. When working with liquid measure, the nurse must subtract the amount of solute from the total desired volume. Consider an example:

Prepare 200 ml of a 10% glycerin solution.

Amount of solute needed for preparation $= x$

Amount of solution desired $= 200$ ml

Percentage concentration of desired solution $= 10$

Percentage concentration of on-hand solute $= 100$

Substituting in the formula gives

$$\frac{x}{200} = \frac{10}{100}$$

Solving for x, we have

$$\frac{x}{200} = \frac{10}{100}$$

$$100x = 2000$$

$$x = \frac{2000}{100}$$

$$x = 20 \text{ ml}$$

The amount of solute needed is 20 ml.
The desired volume in this problem is 200 ml.

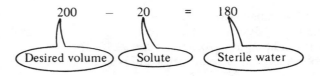

Thus the 20 ml of solute should be added to 180 ml of sterile water to yield 200 ml of solution.

EXAMPLE 7.3

Prepare 400 ml of a 1:50 silver nitrate solution.

1. Amount of solution desired $=$ _____ .
2. Percentage concentration of desired solution $=$ _____ .
3. Percentage concentration of on-hand solute $=$ _____ .
4. Amount of solute needed for preparation $=$ _____ .
5. Substitute the value in the formula.

6. Solve for the amount of solute.

7. How much sterile water should be added to the solute?

Often the desired concentration is expressed in ratio form, as in the last example. It is sometimes necessary to change units of measure in order to solve the problem, as the following example will illustrate.

EXAMPLE 7.4

Prepare 1 qt of a 1:5 hydrogen peroxide solution.

1. Amount of solution desired = _____ . (Use metric units.)
2. Concentration of desired solution = _____ .
3. Concentration of on-hand solute = _____ .
4. Solve for the amount of solute = _____ .

5. How much sterile water should be added to the solute?

SOLUTIONS PREPARED FROM LIQUID SOLUTES WITH CONCENTRATION OTHER THAN 100 PERCENT

Often the solute will be available in concentration other than 100 percent. Solutions are prepared from these solutes in exactly the same manner as in the previous section. In these cases the nurse must use the percentage concentration given on the solute label. Consider the following example: Prepare 1000 ml of a 25% alcohol solution from a 90% alcohol solution.

$$\text{Amount of solute needed for preparation} = x$$

In this case the solute comes from a solution that is on hand.

$$\text{Concentration of desired solution} = 25\%$$

The order is for a 25% alcohol solution.

$$\text{Concentration of on-hand solute} = 90\%$$

The alcohol on hand is in a solution with concentration equal to 90%.

$$\text{Amount of solution desired} = 1000 \text{ ml}$$

Substituting in the formula gives

$$\frac{x}{1000} = \frac{25}{90}$$

Solving for x, we have

$$\frac{x}{1000} = \frac{25}{90}$$

$$90x = 25,000$$

$$x = \frac{25,00\cancel{0}}{9\cancel{0}}$$

$$x = 277.77 = 278 \text{ ml}$$

Therefore 278 ml of the 90% alcohol solute should be used. In order to obtain 1000 ml of solution, since

$$1000 \text{ ml} - 278 \text{ ml} = 722 \text{ ml}$$

722 ml of sterile water should be added to the solute.

EXAMPLE 7.5

Prepare 1 liter of a 3% Lysol solution from a 10% Lysol solution.

1. Amount of solution desired = _____ .
2. Concentration of desired solution = _____ .
3. Concentration of on-hand solute = _____ .
4. Substitute the values in the formula.

5. Solve for the amount of solute.

6. How much sterile water should be mixed with the solute?

If the concentrations are stated in ratio form, the ratio must be converted to a percentage. The next example illustrates a situation where the concentration is stated in ratio form.

EXAMPLE 7.6

Prepare 300 ml of a 1:30 hydrogen peroxide solution from a 1:2 hydrogen peroxide solution.

1. Amount of solution desired = _____ .
2. Concentration of desired solution = _____ .
3. Concentration of on-hand solute = _____ .
4. Solve for the amount of solute.

5. How much sterile water should be mixed with the solute?

Exercise 40

These problems will give you experience in calculations necessary for the preparation of solutions.

1. Prepare 250 ml of 1% sodium chloride solution from a 10% sodium chloride solution.

2. Prepare 250 ml of 2% boric acid solution from boric acid crystals.

3. Prepare 2 liters of 20% sodium bicarbonate solution.

4. Prepare 100 ml of 2% boric acid solution from a 10% boric acid solution.

5. Prepare 500 ml of 10% glycerin solution from liquid glycerin.

6. Prepare 1000 ml of a 10% glucose solution.

7. Prepare 1000 ml of a 1:100 formaldehyde solution from a 50% solution of formaldehyde.

8. Prepare 250 ml of 1:20 glucose solution from crystalline glucose.

9. Prepare 1000 ml of physiologic salt solution (assume 0.9% concentration).

10. Prepare 1000 ml of 1:1000 potassium permanganate solution from 1:100 potassium permanganate solution.

11. Prepare 1000 ml of 1:1000 epinephrine solution from solid epinephrine.

12. Prepare 1 liter of a 2.5% boric acid solution from boric acid crystals.

13. Prepare 500 ml of a 25% cresol solution from a 1:2 solution.

14. Prepare 1000 ml of a 2% vinegar solution.

15. Prepare 2000 ml of a 1:1000 solution of Zephiran.

ANSWERS TO EXAMPLES

Example 7.1

1. 2 oz; change to metric unit of 60 ml
2. 8
3. 100; answer 100% since concentration is not specified.
4. x = grams of crystals

$$\frac{x}{60} = \frac{8}{100}$$

$$100x = 480$$

$$x = \frac{480}{100} = 4.8$$

4.8 g of iodine crystals

Example 7.2

1. 30 ml   2. 10   3. 100
4. $\frac{x}{30} = \frac{10}{100}$

$$100x = 300$$

$$x = \frac{300}{100} = 3$$

3 g of solute used
5. To find how many 10 gr tablets, convert 3 g to grains (1 g = 15 gr)

$$3 \text{ g} = 45 \text{ gr}$$

Each tablet contains 10 gr; thus the nurse uses 4.5 tablets.

Example 7.3

1. 400 ml
2. 2%; use the ratio 1:50 and divide 50 into 1 yielding 0.02. Recall that to change a decimal to a percent, move the decimal two places to the right. Thus 2% is the answer.
3. 100%, assumed
4. x; this is unknown and is in milliliters
5. $\frac{x}{400} = \frac{2}{100}$

6. $\frac{x}{400} = \frac{2}{100}$

$$100x = 800$$

$$x = \frac{800}{100} = 8 \text{ ml}$$

8 ml of solute used.
7. 392 ml, obtained from

$$\begin{array}{r} 400 \text{ ml} \\ -8 \text{ ml} \\ \hline 392 \text{ ml} \end{array}$$

Example 7.4

1. 1000 ml (1 qt = 1000 ml)
2. 20%. A 1:5 concentration is 20%

$$5\overline{)\begin{array}{c}0.20\\1.00\\ \underline{1.00}\end{array}}$$
move the decimal two places
to the right for percent

3. 100%
4. $\frac{x}{1000} = \frac{20}{100}$

   $100x = 20{,}000$

   $x = \frac{20{,}000}{100}$

   $x = 200$ ml

   200 ml of solute used.
5. 800 ml − obtained from

   1000 ml desired
   − 200 ml solute
   800 ml sterile water

Example 7.5

1. 1 liter or 1000 ml
2. 3
3. 10
4. $\frac{x}{1000} = \frac{3}{10}$
5. $\frac{x}{1000} = \frac{3}{10}$

   $10x = 3000$

   $x = \frac{3000}{10}$

   300 ml of solute
6. 700 ml − obtained from

   1000 ml
   − 300 ml
   700 ml

Example 7.6

1. 300 ml
2. 3.33%; 1:30 is 3.33%
3. 50%; 1:2 is 50%
4. $\frac{x}{300} = \frac{3.33}{50}$

   $50x = 999$

   $x = \frac{999}{50} = 19.98$

   $x = 20$ ml, 19.98 is rounded to 20
5. 280 ml, obtained from 300 ml − 20 ml = 280 ml

8 GERIATRIC MEDICATIONS

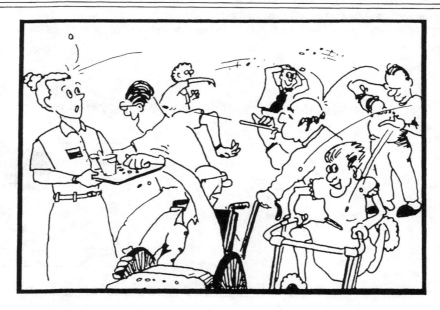

Another pill fight breaks out at the Happy Valley nursing facility.

CHAPTER OBJECTIVES

- Recognize physiologic changes of aging that have implications for the administration of medications
- Solve exercises associated with medications commonly administered to the elderly

INTRODUCTION

The normal physiologic changes of the aging process have many implications for the knowledge and understanding of drug administration in the elderly. Because many elderly patients have chronic illnesses that require more frequent administrations of medication, it is of the utmost importance that nurses be aware of the normal changes associated with aging and the impact of those changes on absorption and excretion of medications. For example, Digoxin is a very common drug administered to the elderly, but it is primarily excreted through the kidneys. Aging decreases the ability of the kidneys to eliminate Digoxin, resulting in high blood levels and more toxicity in the aged. Drug dosages need to be modified for the age-related decreases in renal function, and nurses need to monitor the patient for signs of toxicity as well as all other relevant laboratory data for kidney function.

The elderly client has a decreased total body water and lean body mass while the proportion of body fat increases. The reference for drug dosage may be shifted from age to weight. Because a water-soluble medication is not distributed to fat, more drug remains in the blood and increases chances for toxicity. On the other hand, fat-soluble medications are stored in the body fat, and this increases the accumulation of those drugs.

Gastrointestinal motility slows in the aged, and there is reduced gastric acidity resulting in more erratic rates of dissolving and absorption.

The liver's ability to metabolize medications decreases with aging, which results in longer lasting drug effects, more intense drug effects, and greater incidence of drug toxicity.

The nurse must consistently assess elderly patients for adverse drug reactions, including those side effects that may be mistaken for senility. Communication with the elderly may reveal noncompliance and drug interactions. The nurse can teach and simplify the administration of medications, which may eliminate noncompliance and untoward side effects.

In addition to the physiologic changes altering drug metabolism, drug interactions are a primary concern. The nurse must keep current with all prescription drug information as well as over-the-counter medications that elderly may take.

The following exercise set is designed to provide calculations for drugs commonly administered to the elderly.

Exercise 41

1. The physician orders Oretic 25 mg. How much should the patient receive?

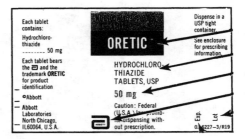

2. The physician orders Lanoxin 0.25 mg. How much should the patient receive?

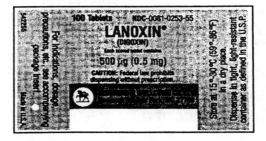

3. The physician orders Morphine 6 mg IM. How much should the patient receive?

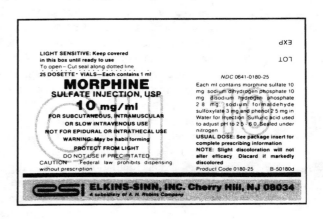

4. The physician orders Lanoxin 0.125 mg. How much should the patient receive?

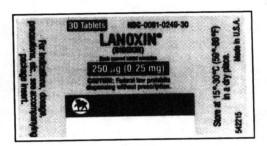

5. The physician orders Nitrostat 0.15 mg prn. How much should the patient receive?

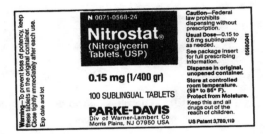

6. The physician orders Pyridium 200 mg. How much should the patient receive?

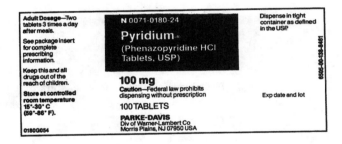

7. The physician orders acetaminophen gr x. How much should the patient receive?

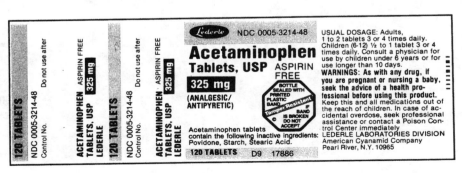

8. The physician orders Decadron 0.25 mg. How much should the patient receive?

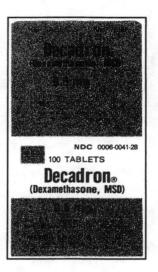

9. The physician orders Aldomet 250 mg. How much should the patient receive?

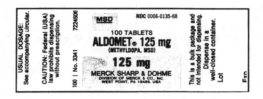

10. The physician orders ferrous sulfate gr v po tid. How much should the patient receive?

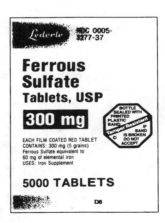

11. The physician orders erythromycin 400 mg. How much should the patient receive?

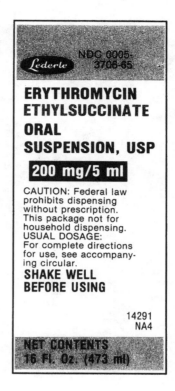

12. The physician orders Benadryl 25 mg. How much should the patient receive?

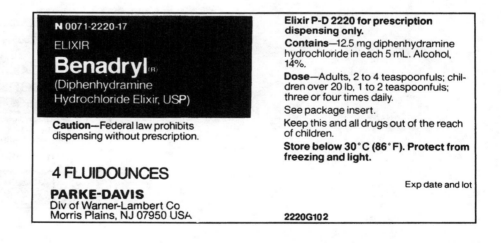

13. The physician orders Kaon Chloride 40 mEq po qd. How much should the patient receive?

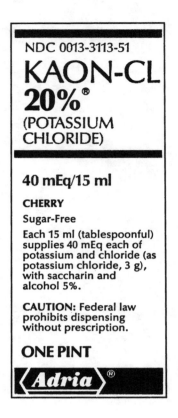

14. The physician orders amoxicillin 250 mg po. How much should the patient receive?

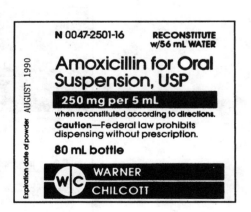

22. The physician orders streptomycin 500 mg. How much should the patient receive?

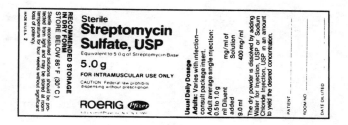

ANSWERS TO TESTS AND EXERCISES

Pretest

1. XVII
2. CCCXLII
3. III
4. XXV
5. 16
6. 257
7. 9
8. 8
9. 17
10. yes
11. no
12. $\frac{3}{16}$
13. $\frac{1}{3}$
14. $\frac{3}{4}$
15. $\frac{11}{56}$
16. $\frac{14}{3}$
17. $\frac{17}{8}$
18. $\frac{133}{10}$
19. $\frac{3}{10}$
20. $\frac{55}{78}$
21. $\frac{4}{3}$
22. $\frac{15}{32}$
23. 5.33
24. $\frac{8}{21}$
25. 0.6
26. 4.047
27. 4.52
28. 7.0993
29. 0.10249
30. 54.4333
31. 0.0325
32. 0.05
33. 0.006
34. 0.89
35. 46%
36. 3%
37. 17.5%
38. 10.5
39. 6
40. 1.909

Exercise 1

1. 3
2. 12
3. 25
4. 19
5. 40
6. 57
7. 20
8. 47
9. 29
10. 200
11. V
12. X
13. XV
14. XLVII
15. VII
16. XXVIII
17. XXXIX
18. LIV
19. CLXXVI
20. DCCXXI
21. 6
22. 25
23. 28
24. 34
25. 79
26. 4
27. 90
28. 95
29. 11
30. 2
31. LXIV
32. LXXXV
33. XIX
34. XXIII
35. XI
36. XCIII
37. XLI
38. LXXVIII
39. LV
40. CXIX
41. 1
42. 3
43. 9
44. 5
45. 13
46. 7
47. 4
48. 8
49. 11
50. 19

Exercise 2

1. $\frac{2}{5}$

2. $\frac{9}{16}$

3. $\frac{7}{8}$

4. $\frac{6}{7}$

5. $\frac{3}{4}$

6. $\frac{2}{3}$

7. $\frac{1}{2}$

8. $\frac{1}{5}$

9. $\frac{1}{2}$

10. $\frac{1}{4}$

11. $\frac{1}{2}$

12. $\frac{1}{5}$

13. $\frac{1}{3}$

14. $\frac{3}{4}$

15. $\frac{3}{16}$

16. $\frac{5}{16}$

17. $\frac{1}{4}$

18. $\frac{4}{5}$

19. $\frac{1}{3}$

20. $\frac{3}{8}$

Exercise 3

1. $\frac{11}{4}$

2. $\frac{3}{2}$

3. $\frac{33}{8}$

4. $\frac{13}{10}$

5. $\frac{29}{8}$

6. $\frac{63}{5}$

7. $\frac{18}{10}$

8. $\frac{19}{3}$

9. $\frac{27}{5}$

10. $\frac{705}{7}$

Exercise 4

1. $\frac{5}{7}$

2. $\frac{1}{4}$

3. $\frac{5}{8}$

4. $\frac{1}{9}$

5. $\frac{17}{15}\left(1\frac{2}{15}\right)$

6. $\frac{3}{22}$

7. $\frac{29}{24}\left(1\frac{5}{24}\right)$

8. $\frac{17}{36}$

9. $4\frac{13}{20}$

10. $\frac{2}{3}$

Exercise 5

1. $\frac{10}{21}$

2. $\frac{3}{8}$

3. $\frac{5}{16}$

4. $\frac{14}{27}$

5. $\frac{1}{10}$

6. $\frac{6}{5}\left(1\frac{1}{5}\right)$

7. $\frac{3}{8}$

8. $\frac{16}{5}\left(3\frac{1}{5}\right)$

9. $\frac{15}{16}$

10. 2

11. $\frac{20}{27}$

12. $\frac{52}{125}$

13. $\frac{9}{22}$

14. $\frac{69}{25}\left(2\frac{19}{25}\right)$

15. $\frac{1}{3}$

16. 6

17. $\frac{105}{2}\left(52\frac{1}{2}\right)$

18. 3

19. $\frac{21}{25}$

20. $\frac{34}{13}\left(2\frac{8}{13}\right)$

Exercise 6

1. $\frac{9}{8}\left(1\frac{1}{8}\right)$

2. 1

3. $\frac{9}{14}$

4. 6

5. $\frac{3}{16}$

6. $\frac{1}{2}$

7. $\frac{1}{18}$

8. $\frac{2}{3}$

9. $\frac{5}{7}$

10. $\frac{11}{26}$

11. $\frac{460}{9}\left(51\frac{1}{9}\right)$

12. $\frac{1}{5}$

13. $\frac{8}{9}$

14. $\frac{49}{2}\left(24\frac{1}{2}\right)$

15. $\frac{1}{2}$

16. $\frac{1}{800}$

17. $\frac{1}{8}$

18. 8

19. $\frac{40}{3}\left(13\frac{1}{3}\right)$

20. $\frac{6}{23}$

Exercise 7

1. 0.75
2. 0.44
3. 0.50
4. 0.23
5. 0.88
6. 0.05
7. 0.60
8. 0.26
9. 0.08
10. 0.66

Exercise 8

1. $\frac{1}{8}$
2. $\frac{2}{5}$
3. $\frac{921}{1000}$
4. $\frac{284}{100}$
5. $\frac{1}{4}$
6. $\frac{1}{50}$
7. $\frac{1}{10}$
8. $\frac{3}{8}$
9. $\frac{3}{4}$
10. $\frac{13}{20}$

Exercise 9

1. 4.271
2. 2.536
3. 1.61
4. 6.418
5. 11.47
6. 34.37
7. 6.32
8. 505.759
9. 1.9935
10. 0.2475

Exercise 10

1. 3.875
2. 0.00988
3. 8.08
4. 5
5. 61.875
6. 3.595
7. 165.11
8. 0.019
9. 0.0125
10. 14

Exercise 11

1. 1.5
2. 4.1
3. 640
4. 6.4
5. 882.55
6. 4.0336
7. 0.17
8. 2400
9. 9.3075
10. 1250

Exercise 12

1. 0.04
2. 0.18
3. 0.005
4. 0.85
5. 0.634
6. 94%
7. 2%
8. 0.7%
9. 84.5%
10. 3.4%

Exercise 13

1. a) $\frac{2 \text{ buses}}{7 \text{ cars}} = \frac{2}{7}$

   b) $\frac{7}{2}$
2. $\frac{8}{11}$
3. $\frac{2}{1}$
4. $\frac{1}{5}$
5. $\frac{18}{1}$

Exercise 14

1. 10
2. 9
3. 0.864
4. 680
5. 100
6. 87500
7. 5
8. 400
9. 16
10. 1
11. 297 miles
12. 10 oranges
13. 30 eggs
14. 20 marbles and 12 marbles
15. $3\frac{1}{3}$ grams
16. 7.5 quarts
17. 5.7 pounds
18. $8\frac{3}{4}$ pounds

Posttest

1. XII
2. V
3. XX
4. XIX
5. II
6. VI
7. 15
8. 4
9. 43
10. 8
11. 30
12. 7
13. denominator
14. yes
15. yes
16. $\frac{3}{16}$
17. $\frac{1}{2}$
18. $\frac{2}{3}$
19. $\frac{14}{39}$
20. $\frac{7}{3}$
21. $\frac{113}{10}$
22. $\frac{109}{5}$
23. $\frac{15}{28}$
24. $\frac{5}{12}$
25. 1
26. $\frac{9}{16}$
27. $\frac{4}{15}$
28. 2.125
29. $\frac{16}{15}$
30. 4
31. 0.8
32. 4.21
33. 2.58
34. 6.908
35. 0.02312
36. 14.42
37. 0.2243
38. 0.05
39. 0.007
40. 0.37
41. 0.012
42. 45%
43. 2%
44. 18.7%
45. 1.25%
46. 9
47. $\frac{21}{11}$
48. 8
49. $1\frac{1}{2}$
50. 10
51. 1

Exercise 15

1. 1 liter
2. 500,000 ml
3. 0.06 liter
4. 8.0 ml
5. 0.025 m
6. 1000 mg
7. 0.25 g
8. 6000 mg
9. 2 kg
10. 3000 m
11. 21.85 m
12. 8450 g
13. 0.03 kl
14. 3000 liters
15. 0.04 kg
16. 0.06 g
17. 0.007 km
18. 250 ml
19. 600,000 liters
20. 0.5 g
21. 140 cm
22. 1 liter
23. 0.01 kg
24. 0.85 m
25. 8,166,000 mm
26. 1020 g

Exercise 16

1. 10 pt
2. 28 fluidrams
3. 256 fluidounces
4. $\frac{3}{4}$ or 0.75 fluidrams

Exercise 17

1. $1\frac{1}{6}$ drams
2. 6720 gr
3. 48 $f\mathfrak{z}$
4. 2700 gr
5. 1.5 gallons
6. 1200 $\mathfrak{m}$
7. $\frac{1}{8}$ or 0.125 $f\mathfrak{z}$
8. 2.5 pt
9. 1.25 $\mathfrak{z}$
10. 12 $\mathfrak{z}$
11. 0.375 $\mathfrak{z}$
12. 896 $f\mathfrak{z}$

Exercise 18

1. 12 t
2. 1.75 glassfuls
3. 1/8 or 0.125 oz
4. 1 T

Exercise 19

1. $\frac{1}{2}$ t
2. 1 glassful
3. 12 t
4. $\frac{1}{2}$ oz
5. 1 oz
6. $\frac{1}{2}$ oz
7. $\frac{2}{3}$ t
8. 240 gtt
9. $\frac{1}{2}$ glassful
10. 2 glassfuls
11. 6 t
12. 6 t
13. 3 T
14. 3 glassfuls
15. 15 gtt

Exercise 20

1. 8 g
2. 45 ml
3. 7.5 mg
4. 45 gtt
5. 1.66 ml
6. 1.5 oz

Exercise 21

1. 3 gr
2. 0.004 g
3. $\frac{1}{2}$ gr
4. 1 g

Exercise 22

1. 15 mg
2. $\frac{1}{240}$ gr
3. 0.2 mg
4. $\frac{1}{20}$ gr

Exercise 23

1. 1 $\mathfrak{z}$
2. 5 $\mathfrak{z}$
3. 90 g
4. 15 g

Exercise 24

1. 11.25 $\mathfrak{m}$
2. 1 ml
3. 13.5 $\mathfrak{m}$
4. 2 ml

Exercise 25

1. 3000 ml
2. $\frac{5}{6}$ $\mathfrak{z}$
3. 30 ml
4. 5 $\mathfrak{z}$

Exercise 26

1. 6.6 lb
2. 9.1 kg
3. 30.8 lb
4. 24.3 kg
5. 53.5 lb
6. 17 kg

Exercise 27

1. 59 F
2. 28 C
3. 37.4 F
4. 20 C
5. 98.6 F
6. −10 C

Exercise 28

1. 15 $\mathfrak{m}$
2. 105 gr
3. 14 T
4. $\frac{5}{6}$ gr
5. 1500 ml
6. 480 g
7. 1.6 ml
8. 2 g
9. 10 mg
10. 1.33 or $1\frac{1}{3}$ ml
11. $1\frac{2}{3}$ $\mathfrak{z}$
12. 30 gtt
13. $\frac{1}{15}$ gr
14. 22.5 mg
15. $3\frac{1}{3}$ $\mathfrak{z}$
16. 75 gr
17. 30 g
18. 3 $\mathfrak{z}$
19. 2.5 $\mathfrak{z}$
20. 60 gr
21. 6 $\mathfrak{m}$
22. 60 ml
23. $\frac{3}{4}$ gr
24. 7.5 $\mathfrak{m}$
25. 10 C
26. 44.6 F
27. 28.4 F
28. 38.9 C
29. 37 C
30. 12.2 F

Exercise 29

1. 5 ml

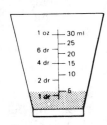

2. 11.4 ml
3. 10 ml

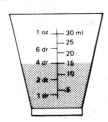

4. One tablet
5. 15 ml

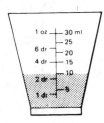

6. 6.8 ml
7. 2 tablets
8. 10 ml

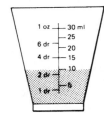

9. 1 tablet
10. 10 ml
11. 5.0 ml
12. 2 tablets
13. 0.6 ml
14. $\frac{1}{2}$ tablet
15. 2 tablets
16. 2 tablets
17. 2 tablets
18. 1 capsule
19. 1 tablet
20. 9 ml
21. 2 tablets
22. $\frac{1}{2}$ tablet
23. 4 ml
24. 2 tablets
25. $\frac{1}{2}$ tablet
26. 2 ml

Exercise 30

1. 3 tablets
2. 1 tablet
3. $\frac{1}{2}$ tablet
4. $\frac{1}{2}$ tablet
5. $\frac{1}{2}$ tablet
6. 4 ml
7. 2 tablets
8. $2\frac{1}{2}$ tablets
9. 2 tablets
10. 3 ml
11. 2.5 ml
12. 2.5 ml

Exercise 31

1. 1.5 ml
2. 1.6 ml

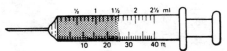

3. 0.3 ml

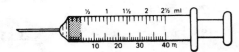

4. 1 ml
5. 0.8 ml or 12 ♏

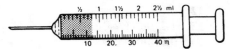

6. $\frac{1}{2}$ ml

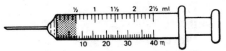

7. $\frac{1}{2}$ ml
8. 2.2 ml

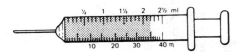

9. 1 ml

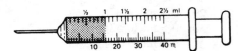

10. 0.9 ml or 14 ♏

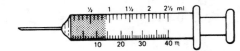

Exercise 32

1. $\frac{1}{2}$ ml
2. 2 ml
3. 0.4 ml or 6 ℳ
4. 1.5 ml
5. $\frac{1}{2}$ ml
6. 1.5 ml
7. 1.5 ml
8. $\frac{1}{2}$ ml
9. 0.25 ml or 4 ℳ
10. 0.8 ml (0.75)
11. 0.7 ml (0.67)
12. 0.9 ml
13. 1.2 ml (1.25)
14. 0.8 ml (0.75)
15. 1.2 ml (1.25)
16. 1.5 ml (1.52)
17. 0.2 ml
18. 1.2 ml (1.25)
19. 0.5 ml
20. 0.4 ml
21. 0.7 ml (0.67)
22. 1 ml
23. 0.5 ml
24. 0.2 ml (0.25)
25. 0.2 ml (0.25)
26. 0.5 ml
27. 0.5 ml
28. 0.5 ml (0.47)
29. 0.4 ml (0.375)
30. 0.5 ml (0.53)
31. 0.3 ml (0.28)
32. 2 ml
33. 1 ml
34. 0.5 ml
35. 0.5 ml

Exercise 33

1. 1.2 ml

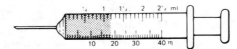

2. 2 ml

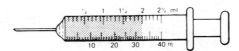

3. 35 U

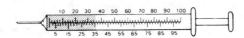

4. 1.5 ml

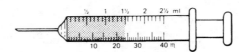

5. 1.2 ml

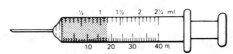

6. 0.8 ml (0.75)
7. 1.3 ml
8. 16 U

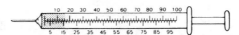

9. 19 U

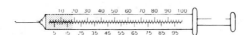

10. 0.8 ml

Exercise 34

1. 2.5 ml
   330 mg/ml
   1.5 ml
2. 3.4 ml
   250 mg/ml
   1 ml
   0.6 ml
3. 6.6 ml
   250 mg/ml
   1.4 ml
4. 4 ml
   0.5 g/2.2 ml
   1.1 ml
5. 1.25 ml
6. 2.7 ml
   250 mg/1.5 ml
   3 ml
7. 9.0 ml
   400 mg/ml
   1.25 ml
8. 10 ml
9. 1.8 ml
   500 mg/ml
   1 ml
10. 7.0 ml
    1 g/2.0 ml
    2 ml
11. 10 ml
12. 10 ml
13. 10 ml
14. 1.1 ml
15. 0.9 ml

Exercise 35

1. 7 gtt/min
2. 14 gtt/min
3. 21 gtt/min
4. 83 gtt/min
5. 42 gtt/min
6. 10 gtt/min
7. 31 gtt/min
8. 21 gtt/min
9. 42 gtt/min

Exercise 36

1. 5 hours
2. 4 hours
3. 7 hours 8 minutes
4. 3 hours 45 minutes
5. 5 hours 33 minutes
6. 3 hours 20 minutes
7. 2 hours 40 minutes
8. 12 hours 30 minutes
9. 4 hours

Exercise 37

1. 17 gtt/min
2. 50 gtt/min
3. 100 gtt/min
4. 100 gtt/min
5. 17 gtt/min
6. 25 gtt/min
7. 100 gtt/min
8. 33 gtt/min
9. 25 gtt/min

Exercise 38

1. 20 mg
2. 4 mg
3. (a) 7 mg
   (b) 23 mg
4. 1.3 gr
5. 4 mg
6. (a) 2 mg
   (b) 4 mg
7. 20 mg
8. 15 mg
9. 100 mg
10. 184 mg
11. 120,000 U
12. 67 mg
13. 3 mg
14. 0.5 mg
15. 40 mg
16. 0.27 mg
17. 16.7 mg
18. 6.67 mg
19. 66.7 mg
20. 0.1 mg
21. 66 mg
22. 6.5 mg
23. 14 mg

Exercise 39

1. 62.5 mg per dose
   (125 mg per day)
2. 416.7 mg per dose
   (2500 mg per day)
3. 150 mg per dose
   (450 mg per day)
4. 187.5 mg per dose
   (750 mg per day)
5. 180 mg per dose
   (360 mg per day)
6. 72 mg per dose
   (288 mg per day)
7. 166.7 mg per dose
   (1000 mg per day)

Exercise 40

1. 25 ml solute
   225 ml sterile water
2. 5 g solute
   250 ml solution
3. 400 g solute
   1600 ml sterile water
4. 20 ml solute
   80 ml sterile water
5. 50 ml solute
   450 ml sterile water
6. 100 g solute
   dilute to 1000 ml mark
7. 20 ml solute
   980 ml sterile water
8. 12.5 g solute
   dilute to 250 ml mark
9. 9 g solute
   dilute to 1000 ml mark
10. 100 ml solute
    900 ml sterile water
11. 1 g solute
    dilute to 1000 ml mark
12. 25 g solute
    dilute to 1000 ml mark
13. 250 ml solute
    250 ml sterile water
14. 20 ml solute
    980 ml sterile water
15. 2 ml solute
    1998 ml sterile water

Exercise 41

1. $\frac{1}{2}$ tablet
2. $\frac{1}{2}$ tablet
3. 0.6 ml
4. $\frac{1}{2}$ tablet
5. 1 tablet
6. 2 tablets
7. 2 tablets
8. $\frac{1}{2}$ tablet
9. 2 tablets
10. 1 tablet
11. 10 ml
12. 10 ml
13. 15 ml
14. 5 ml
15. 0.6 ml
16. 0.2 ml
17. 1 ml
18. $\frac{1}{2}$ ml
19. 0.7 ml
20. 4 ml
21. 2.5 ml
22. 1.25 ml

INDEX